Praise for *LIVING WELL WITH BACK PAIN*

"The authors *empower* patients to take charge of their back pain and choose the therapy most suitable to them. The book is cutting-edge and easy to follow while being in-depth and encyclopedic—covering both somatic and psychological aspects of low back pain."
—Alex Vaasen, NLP, senior staff and quality co-coordinator, Department of Physiotherapy, Leiden Medical Center, Leiden, the Netherlands

"As a spine surgeon with over thirty-five years of experience in treating patients with back pain, I appreciate what Drs. Winter and Bach have done for back pain sufferers by writing this book. It is particularly helpful for patients in how to take charge of their own health care destiny, how to select a doctor, and how to access quality information about back pain from the Internet. I will definitely recommend it to my patients."
— Mark D. Brown, MD, PhD, professor and chairman, Department of Orthopaedics and Rehabilitation, Leonard M. Miller School of Medicine, University of Miami

"The information is sound and clearly presented for patient use. I will plan on recommending this book for my patients with back pain. The information is scientifically sound and is written by one of the giants of spinal care, Dr. Robert Winter."
—Dale E. Rowe, MD

"Drs. Winter and Bach provide vital information that is easily understandable by lay persons, but should also be read by any health care professional who routinely treats individuals with disorders of the spine. . . . I strongly recommend this to anyone who has back pain, has had back pain, or wants to learn about ways to avoid back pain in the future."
—William C. Lauerman, MD, Georgetown University Hospital, Department of Orthopaedics

"Doctors Winter and Bach both have extensive experience in the evaluation and treatment of back pain, and this book provides comprehensive information regarding the various evidence-based treatment options available for the patient suffering from back pain. . . . [It] will guide them into appropriate treatment pathways and help avoid unproven, misleading choices."
—Thomas G. Lowe, MD, clinical professor, Orthopaedics, University of Colorado Health Sciences Center, Woodridge Spine Center, PC

"As a nutritional counselor who has worked for over twenty-five years with people suffering from chronic illnesses, I am keenly aware of the toll that back problems take on their lives. Drs. Winter, Bach, and the Twin Cities Spine Center present a reader-friendly, comprehensive guide that will prove invaluable for persons with back pain. Its focus on self-care as the foundation of the unique Back Care Pyramid empowers the patient to view herself as the lead participant in her own healing. Kudos to the authors for highlighting the pivotal role of nutrition for healing and maintaining back health."

> —Darlene Kvist, MS, CNS, LN, director, Nutritional Weight and Wellness, Saint Paul, Minnesota

"*Living Well with Back Pain* is unique in breadth and scope. The most advanced and scientifically sound mind-body techniques for coping with pain and healing quickly are highlighted—empowering the patient to take charge of his own back health."

> —Alfred Messore, MD, psychiatrist, American Board of Psychiatry and Neurology; former program director, Washington, DC, Psychiatric Society

"Very well written . . . easy to read and covers *everything*. I wish I had had [this book] before my surgery."   —Arlyne Selvestra, back pain patient

"[E]xtremely comprehensive, easy to read, and . . . full of important information and references. . . . [T]he 'back bible' of our time."

> —Patricia Brahm, back pain patient

"A must-have resource for anyone who is experiencing back pain or who is considering surgery . . . comprehensive and informative. Having had three back surgeries myself . . . I would not hesitate to recommend this book to anyone."

> —Lisette Wright, back pain patient

"This is a very comprehensive book about back pain that covers all aspects of treatment, from alternative approaches to complex surgical treatments . . . clearly written and easily understandable."

> —Leon Root, MD, Department of Orthopaedic Surgery, Hospital for Special Surgery

"A comprehensive guide to the many treatment options available. Written by professionals in a language simple and understandable enough for laypeople to appreciate, this book will be a welcome addition to the body of literature on this important subject."

> —Janice T. Sacks, vice chair, Scoliosis Association, Inc.

LIVING WELL WITH

Back Pain

What Your Doctor

Doesn't Tell You . . .

That You Need to Know

ROBERT B. WINTER, MD
MARILYN L. BACH, PhD
and The Twin Cities Spine Center

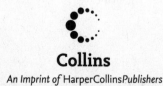

Collins
An Imprint of HarperCollins*Publishers*

Illustrations in Chapters 1, 2, 4, and 17, and the illustration on the bottom of page 248 in Chapter 21 © Peter Lane.

Photography in Chapters 19 and 21 © John Lehn.

FIRST EDITION

Designed by Joy O'Meara

Library of Congress Cataloging-in-Publication Data

Winter, Robert B., 1932–
 Living well with back pain: what your doctor doesn't tell you . . . that you need to know / by Robert B. Winter, Marilyn L. Bach, and the Twin Cities Spine Center.
  p. cm.
 Includes bibliographical references and index.
 ISBN-13: 978-0-06-079227-5
 ISBN-10: 0-06-079227-2
 1. Backache. 2. Backache—Treatment. 3. Self-care, Health.
I. Bach, Marilyn L. II. Title.

 RD768.W538 2006
 617.5'64—dc22

               2006041072

06 07 08 09 10 WB/RRD 10 9 8 7 6 5 4 3 2 1

MEDICAL DISCLAIMER

This book contains advice and information relating to health care. It is not intended to replace medical advice and should be used to supplement rather than replace regular care by your doctor. It is recommended that you seek your physician's advice before embarking on any medical program or treatment. All efforts have been made to assure the accuracy of the information contained in this book as of the date of publication. The publisher and the authors disclaim liability for any medical outcomes that may occur as a result of applying the methods suggested in this book.

CONTENTS

Acknowledgments   ix

Introduction

Why You Need This Book   1

1 The Good News about Back Pain   7

2 Where Does Back Pain Come From,
   and Why Do I Hurt?   10

3 Nonsurgical Treatments   36

4 Surgical Treatments   56

5 The Twenty-Five Most Common Questions
   about Back Pain and Its Treatment   70

6 Adopting the Right Mindset   77

7 The Benefits of Taking Charge and the Costs
   of Being Passive   86

8 Self-Care   100

9 Using the Internet   104

10 Face-to-Face with Your Family Physician   109

11 Tests   119

12 Step-by-Step: Using the Back Care Pyramid   125

13 Choosing the Right Treatment   136

14 Dealing with Your Health Insurance   141

15 Face-to-Face with the Physical Therapist 163

16 Face-to-Face with the Medical Specialists 180

17 Taking Control When You Need Surgery 195

18 The Mind–Body Connection 213

19 Recovering Quickly and Safely After Surgery 222

20 How Do I Get Back to Work? 231

21 Keeping Your Back Healthy and Strong 237

22 What Do I Do If My Surgery
Doesn't Seem to Have Worked? 276

23 Back Pain in Children and Adolescents 282

Appendix A: Resources 289

Appendix B: Glossary 307

Appendix C: References 319

Index 337

ACKNOWLEDGMENTS

Many people have made substantial contributions to the development of this book. We thank Lorie Schleck, MA, PT, who provided technical and writing support and edited the entire draft manuscript. Special thanks to Scott Edlestein, literary consultant, who insightfully shepherded this project from beginning to end. We thank Linda Konner, literary agent, for successfully linking this effort to the HarperCollins *Living Well* series.

Members of the Twin Cities Spine Center, Minneapolis and Saint Paul, provided the backbone of this effort. Ron Anderson, administrator, facilitated the work of multiple contributors, adding patience and humor through the hills and valleys of this endeavor. We thank the surgeons of the Twin Cities Spine Center, Julie Abnet, RN, Lisa Butler, RN, and Cate Pandiscio, PT, PA-C, for their review and critique, and Doug Toft, writer and editor, Minneapolis, Minnesota.

Special acknowledgment to Lyla Westrup, education coordinator, for her tireless administrative assistance and coordination of the work. Stacy Claassen, education/research liaison, provided helpful administrative assistance.

We thank Janice T. Sacks, vice chair of the Scoliosis Association, Inc., senior editor of *Backtalk,* and past president of the Scoliosis Association, Inc., for her insightful and helpful commentary on the entire manuscript.

Dr. Bach wishes to thank Alice Erickson for her patient and highly competent research and editorial assistance.

We thank the editorial staff of HarperCollins, Sarah Durand and Jeremy Cesarec.

The illustrations are by Peter Lane, St. Paul, Minnesota; photography by John Lehn and modeling by Kristin Smith, KAS Fitness Training, Minneapolis, Minnesota.

Introduction

Why You Need This Book

by Joseph Perra, MD, of the Twin Cities Spine Center

Chances are you're reading this book because your back hurts—perhaps badly—and you're not sure what to do about it.

You're not alone. Back problems are among the top ten most common ailments that people live with. More than 80% of all American adults suffer from frequent or chronic back pain at some point in their lives. Most of these people have no clue about what they need to get better. Should they have surgery? Do yoga? Exercise more? Will massage help? Can they trust a chiropractor? And of all these options, which ones will their insurance cover?

Here's the good news: More than 95% of those with acute back pain can be cured without surgery. In fact, 80% of all people with acute back pain can recover fully without seeing a doctor, chiropractor, or other health care professional. In this book you will also find out when to see a doctor as an emergency.

Now for the bad news: Whatever the cause of your back pain, the wrong treatment could make your bad back much, much worse. Making the wrong treatment decisions or choosing the wrong health care professional could cause you big trouble (see Chapter 7).

You can't afford to let others make your health care decisions for

1

you. You need to pick your own health care professionals carefully. You need to know what questions to ask, when to ask them, and whom to ask. You need to know about your choices and options in advance so that you are knowledgeable enough to make the right decisions. And you need to know when to say yes to a suggested treatment, when to say no, and when to ask for more information (and possibly a second opinion).

In short, in order to heal your back as quickly, completely, and safely as possible, *you need to become your own best health care advocate*. No one else can do this for you. Other people can and will help, but *you* must make all the most important decisions and choices. This book will show you how to make the right ones.

Living Well with Back Pain is designed to help you understand your back, ask the right questions, get the right medical professionals on your side, and do the right things at the right times. It has been written with three essential goals in mind: (1) helping you get the best treatment, (2) helping you choose the best and most appropriate health care professionals, and (3) advising you on how to enjoy the fastest recovery. You will be introduced to the Back Care Pyramid, a step-by-step guide to the complexities of back care options. You will learn exactly what to do every step of the way to make sure that you get what you need from the people who are most qualified to provide it. You will learn what to say and do to minimize the chance of something going wrong.

Because each person's back is unique, *there is no one-size-fits-all treatment for back pain*. Your back must be carefully examined by a properly qualified and appropriate professional, and any treatment must be custom-crafted to suit your unique combination of body type, health history, type and intensity of pain, lifestyle, age, gender, and diagnosis. With some attention and effort, you can dramatically increase your chances for a fast and full recovery from back pain.

We do not offer simplistic (and potentially damaging) solutions. Instead, you will read about the most up-to-date evidence-based medicine that has been scientifically proven to heal your back better than a placebo and better than your body can heal itself. You can feel confident that we will not recommend any treatment for you that has not been proven effective.

We will help you pick the right professionals to get an accurate diagnosis. With the right people, you can then create the very best treatment for your own back, body, and personality. This book offers a user-friendly guide to your insurance options—a sine qua non in today's medical world and a topic not commonly addressed by other back books. (Treatment information for children and adolescents is included in Chapter 23.)

Living Well with Back Pain will guide you through the maze of information, tests, diagnoses, and options for treatment. In down-to-earth language, it will

- Explain all the many different causes of lumbar and thoracic back pain. (We have chosen not to address issues involving the neck, a very complex topic best left for another book.)
- Help you understand what works, what doesn't, and why.
- Show you what you can do to reduce or eliminate your back pain *on your own*.
- Outline and explain each different test for the causes of back pain.
- Explain what each potential diagnosis means and what your treatment options are for each one.
- Offer a comprehensive approach to treatment, with surgery being neither "the answer" nor the "course of last resort."
- Enable you to pick the right health care professionals for you and your unique situation.
- Explain exactly what questions and requests to bring to each professional.
- Give you all the tools you need to heal as quickly and effectively as possible.

- Take the fear and mystery out of back pain treatment.
- Show you how to keep your back strong and healthy after successful treatment.

In short, this book is your single best tool for healing, treating, and taking care of your back—and for becoming your back's #1 health advocate.

Why should you read this book and pay attention to us? We offer a unique collaboration of experts: patient and wellness professional Marilyn Bach, physical therapist Lorie Schleck, and spine surgeon Robert Winter, all supported by an internationally renowned medical institution. The Twin Cities Spine Center, with locations in Minneapolis and St. Paul, is one of the world's largest and most respected centers for the diagnosis and treatment of back problems. Dr. Robert Winter is a renowned spine surgeon, clinical professor of orthopedic surgery at the University of Minnesota, and a research consultant to the Twin Cities Spine Center. He has successfully treated thousands of people for back pain, both surgically and nonsurgically, during a forty-year career. Dr. Marilyn Bach is a health and fitness writer, a wellness consultant whose clients include the 3M Company and the University of Rhode Island, a former faculty member of the University of Minnesota and University of Wisconsin Medical Schools, and the coauthor of the popular book *ShapeWalking: Six Easy Steps to Your Best Body*.

But it is more than just expertise that brought Bob, Marilyn, Lorie, and me together. In 2001, Marilyn began experiencing severe lower back pain that left her unable to work or exercise and barely able to walk. Knowing how harmful improper treatment could be, she developed an approach to taking charge of her own back care and becoming her own ideal back advocate. Using this process, she selected me as her surgeon, and I operated on her successfully.

Afterward, working together, the two of us designed a back recovery plan uniquely suited for Marilyn. By following this plan,

Marilyn returned her back to complete health only seven weeks after her surgery—an astonishingly fast recovery.

After some discussions with Bob Winter, we realized that what worked for Marilyn—a combination of the careful selection of health care professionals, custom-tailored treatment and recovery, and assertive consumer advocacy—could work for anyone with back pain, potentially benefiting millions of people. Thus, this book was born.

Everything your back needs for the fastest, safest, and most effective healing is right here. So simply turn the page, and begin taking charge of your bad back.

1

The Good News about Back Pain

We begin with three pieces of very good news:

1. *Acute back pain is one of the most common health problems.* In fact, 80% of all adults have (or will have) at least one episode of moderate to severe back pain. Why is this good news? Because it means medical science has extensively studied back pain and knows a lot about it.

It also means you're not alone. Millions of people have probably had the exact same problem you do and have healed successfully. With a little careful searching, you can find a medical professional who is very familiar with your specific problem and who has had repeated success in treating people for it.

2. *Most back pain doesn't require any professional medical treatment at all.* Most cases of back pain are healed naturally by the body and thus go away on their own in a few hours or days. You don't need to see your family doctor, a chiropractor, or a physical therapist (let alone an orthopedic surgeon or a neurosurgeon).

3. *You can treat most back pain successfully yourself.* Just do these simple things and there's an 80% chance that your back will be better in a few hours to a few days:

- *Take it easy. Avoid heavy lifting and high-impact activity (jogging, tennis, golf, volleyball, etc.).*
- *Avoid prolonged sitting. If necessary, do some of your work standing up, or take a ten-minute standing or walking break each hour.*
- *Put ice on the painful area of your back during the first twenty-four hours of pain, then heat thereafter.*
- *Take an over-the-counter pain medication such as aspirin or acetaminophen (Tylenol), or an antiinflammatory medication such as naproxen sodium (Aleve) or ibuprofen (Advil).*
- *Do not spend a week in bed.*
- *Rest frequently in the contour position, which is illustrated in the figure.*

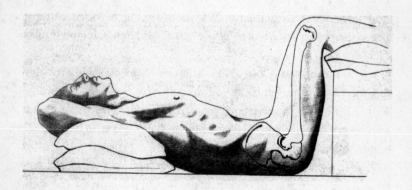

Figure 1: The contour position. The hips and knees are bent to almost 90 degrees in order to fully relax the spine and the strong flexor muscles.

Because most back pain is benign and goes away on its own, there's usually no point in spending time and money on expensive doctor visits and tests. However, there are several circumstances in which you should *immediately* see a medical professional:

- If the pain is so severe that you can't sleep or function at all
- If you lose control of muscles in your leg(s)
- If you lose control of your bladder or bowels

Here's the happy paradox: Many people buy this book, read this chapter, and follow its advice. As a result, they get better without seeing a doctor, save themselves the cost of a health appointment, and never need to read any of the remaining chapters. If this happens to you, that's great! But if you are one of the 20% of back pain sufferers who need more help, read on. All the information and support you need are here.

2

Where Does Back Pain Come From, and Why Do I Hurt?

Understanding your back pain begins with a basic look at how the spine looks, how it works, and what can go wrong.

■ What the Spine Looks Like and How It Works

The spine is a complex structure. It performs several vital functions:

1. Supporting the weight of the trunk so that you can sit and walk upright.
2. Permitting trunk motion so that you can bend to tie your shoes.
3. Protecting the spinal cord (a structure that runs down from the brain and supplies nerves to the arms, chest, legs, and internal organs). Injury to the spinal cord can lead to paralysis.

The spine is a column of twenty-four bones called vertebrae. Seven of these vertebrae are in the neck (cervical vertebrae), twelve are in the chest (thoracic vertebrae), and five are in the lower back (lumbar vertebrae). The sacrum sits at the base of the spine and is part of the pelvis.

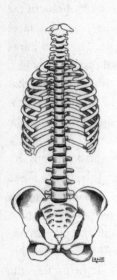

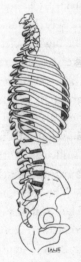

Figure 2a: A frontal view of the whole spine and pelvis. There are seven cervical (neck), twelve thoracic (chest area with ribs attached), and five lumbar (lower back) vertebrae. The sacrum is at the base of the spine and is part of the pelvis.

Figure 2b: A side view of a normal spine. The cervical (neck) and lumbar (lower back) vertebrae are in lordosis (a curve with the apex forward), and the thoracic (chest area) vertebrae are in kyphosis (a curve with the apex backward).

The disc is a firm, rubbery cushion that sits between the front (or body) of two vertebrae. Because it is compressible, the disc allows the spine to move in several directions. It also absorbs vertical loads such as the jarring your spine feels if you suddenly sit down hard.

The center of the disc is gel-like. The outside is a tough wall called the annulus fibrosis (often shortened to annulus). The annulus is thicker and therefore stronger in some areas than in others. The annulus has small nerve fibers, but the center of the disc does not.

Along the back of the spine are small joints called facet (fuh-set) joints. These joints are formed by parts of adjacent vertebrae. In the lumbar spine, the upper vertebra forms the inner part of a facet joint while the lower vertebra forms the outer part. The facet joints allow for spine motion and help protect the spinal cord.

In the chest area, the ribs attach to the spine with little joints that allow the ribs to move up and down as we breathe in and out. Ligaments are important supporting structures. They run along the front, side, and back of the spine and add stability.

Several muscles control spine movement. The most obvious are the big muscles that run up and down the center of the back. These are called extensor muscles because they help extend the trunk (bend it backward). Beneath the extensors are the multifidi, a group of smaller muscles that help rotate the trunk and play an important role in dynamically stabilizing the spine. The psoas is a big muscle in front of the lumbar spine and hips. It helps flex the trunk (bend it forward) and flex the hips (bringing the knee toward the chest).

The abdominal muscles play an important role in spine function. They stabilize the trunk, preventing unwanted motion. They also rotate and flex the trunk. Several muscles make up the abdominal—or "abs"—muscle group:

1. The rectus abdominus is the most central muscle of the group. It runs from the chest to the pelvis.
2. The internal and external obliques run diagonally to the rectus abdominus.
3. The transversalis is a deep central muscle.
4. The quadratus lumborum is a deep posterior muscle.

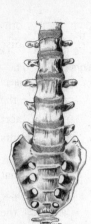

Figure 3a: A frontal view of the lumbar spine and sacrum. Each vertebra is separated from the next by a disc (intervertebral disc) that has a tough outer layer called the annulus fibrosis (cross-hatched areas). The sacrum is a single bone with holes in it where the nerves come out.

Figure 3b: A posterior (looking from the back) view of the lumbar spine and sacrum. In between each vertebra are ligaments that strengthen the spine and protect the nerves. The ligamentum flavum has fibers running up and down the center of the spine, and there are facet joints where each vertebra comes in contact with the next. The facet joints also have strengthening ligaments (the capsular ligaments or capsules).

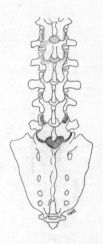

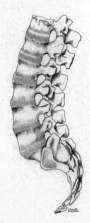

Figure 3c: A side view of the lumbar spine and sacrum. The vertebrae are lined up in lordosis ("sway-back") and are separated from each other by the discs. In the back are the spinous processes, which are the "bumps" you can feel when you touch your back.

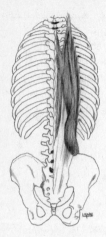

Figure 4a: A view of the back of the spine showing the large muscles running up and down. These are the long extensors of the spine, which are critical for stabilization and backward bending.

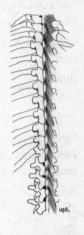

Figure 4b: A view of the back of the spine showing the short, deep muscles responsible for segmental stabilization and rotation.

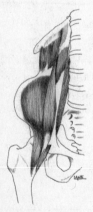

Figure 4c: A view of the deep muscles in the front of the lumbar spine and pelvis. These are responsible for spine and hip flexion.

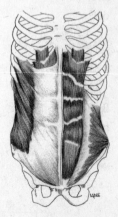

Figure 4d: A view of the muscles of the abdominal wall. In the center are the abs, and off to the side are the obliques and the tranversalis muscles.

Nerves run from the spinal cord to various body structures through openings in the spine called foraminae. As we shall see later, it is very important that the foraminae remain open for these nerves to function properly.

In the thoracic spine, nerves run along the ribs to the intercostal muscles (the muscles between the ribs), which allow us to move our ribs up and down as we breathe. In the lumbar spine, nerves go out to the legs, bowel, and bladder, controlling the movement and function of these structures. The nerves that control movement and function are called motor nerves. When a motor nerve is affected, you might experience muscle weakness in the legs or disrupted bowel or bladder function. Sensory nerves run from the legs, bowel, and bladder to the spinal cord and up to the brain. They register pain, touch, and other sensations. If you step on a sharp stone, the sensory nerves send a pain signal to the brain. Sensory nerves also tell the brain when your bladder is full. When sensory nerves are affected, you might experience numbness in the legs or an inability to sense a full bladder.

During your back examination, the medical specialist will check for motor nerve problems by testing your leg muscle strength. He or she will also check for sensory nerve problems by looking for areas of numbness.

▎ What Can Go Wrong

Back pain can come from many different parts of the back and even from places outside the spine. Once your doctor finds the source of your back pain, he or she will give you a diagnosis. In this section we will describe common back diagnoses: what they are, what causes them, what you might feel or experience with a certain diagnosis, and how a given diagnosis might be treated.

Muscle and Ligament Strains and Sprains

What is it?

Just like our knee and shoulder joints, the spine can suffer a strain or sprain. These conditions occur when muscles or ligaments in your back are overloaded or stressed. A strain is a pulled muscle, and a sprain is a pulled ligament.

What causes it?

Strains and sprains are most often caused by lifting or twisting. For example, you might strain your lower back by carrying a heavy suitcase or picking up a heavy package. Minor falls and other injuries can also cause this problem. Major trauma such as an automobile accident or a fall from a significant height can cause complete ligament tears or ruptures, which can be seen on X-rays, CT (computed tomography) scans, or MRI (magnetic resonance imaging) scans. Strains and sprains cannot be detected with these techniques.

What does it feel like?

Pain in the injured area is the main symptom of a back sprain or strain. You will have muscle tightness and soreness, but you will not have pain in the legs.

Muscle strains can become a chronic (long-lasting) problem if the cause is not addressed. For example, a woman with large breasts may have chronic upper back muscle strain. In this situation, breast reduction may be a way to diminish muscle strain and relieve back pain. Chronic bad posture can also cause muscle strain. This can be corrected with proper exercise and good posture training.

How might it be treated?

Most muscle strains and sprains resolve themselves in a few days without any specific treatment.

Disc Herniation

What is it?

Almost everyone has heard of a ruptured or herniated disc. This occurs when the outside part of the disc (the annulus) ruptures and the central part of the disc seeps out or herniates. A partial tear of the annulus causes only back pain. A complete tear of the annulus can cause the ruptured disc material to press against the spinal cord (rare) or on the spinal nerves (much more common). Pressure on the spinal nerves causes acute back pain and acute leg pain going down below the knee. The diagnosis of disc herniation is best made by MRI examination.

What causes it?

Usually but not always a sudden stressful load causes disc herniation. For example, Dr. Winter suffered a disc herniation when he lifted a heavy patient by himself. Mrs. Winter suffered a disc herniation from violent vomiting due to a kidney stone. Disc herniations are most common in the 30- to 50-year age group (though they can occur in teenagers). Disc herniations are less common after age 50, as the discs naturally dry up and are no longer prone to rupture.

What does it feel like?

Pressure on the nerve can vary from mild to severe; consequently, the symptoms can vary in severity, too. With a more severe disc herniation, you may have numbness in the leg or foot, muscle weakness, and changes in your reflexes (which your doctor will check with a reflex hammer). With smaller herniations, you may feel only back pain.

Sometimes a very large central disc herniation (where the middle part of the disc ruptures) can cause a loss in bowel and bladder function along with numbness in the genital area (called cauda equina syndrome). Emergency lower back surgery is indicated in this situation. Emergency surgery is also necessary if a thoracic disc rupture causes paralysis.

How might it be treated?

Most disc herniations are treated nonsurgically. When your pain is acute (indicative of a recent injury), pain medications including narcotics may be necessary. Spasms in the back muscles are common with this condition and can be treated with heat or cold, whichever one you respond to best. Resting on your back with your hips and knees flexed (the contour position) can be most comfortable and beneficial (see Fig. 1, p. 8).

In a few days, your symptoms should subside. In this subacute phase, you should be up and about, not lying in bed. Pain medications are reduced, with narcotics no longer indicated. Lifting should be avoided, but active walking is encouraged. If available, swimming pool exercises can help, since the buoyancy of the water decreases stress on the spine. Early on, simply walking and moving in the pool are best. As you feel better, you can start swimming laps or try a water aerobics class.

As you heal, you may experience periodic episodes of increased pain. Do not panic. This is normal. Go back to the tried-and-true principles of self-care: rest in the contour position, use ice or heat, avoid heavy lifting and repeated bending. After a few days of good self-care, your symptoms should subside.

Some people with disc herniations do require surgery. If your pain is severe and intolerable and does not go away even with strong narcotic medicine, or if you have significant weakness in the foot or leg that does not go away in a few days to a week or two, then surgery may very well be necessary.

One thing you should try to avoid is continued use of narcotic medications such as morphine, Demerol (meperidine), Oxycontin (oxycodone), and codeine. Along with posing a risk for addiction, these medications can cause you bodily harm, especially respiratory and digestive depression.

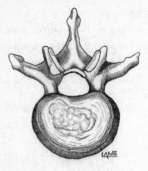

Figure 5a: This is a cross-sectional view of a lumbar disc. The outer layers are the tough annulus fibrosis; the softer, cushioning nucleus pulposis is in the center. The artist has shown a mild protrusion of the central nucleus into but not through the annulus. This is commonly known as an internal disc derangement or annular tear.

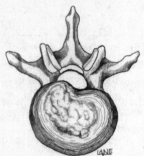

Figure 5b: Here we see a more significant penetration of the disc material partway through the annulus with a bulging of the disc into the spinal canal. This is typically called a bulging disc.

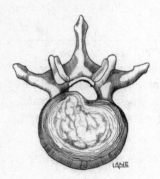

Figure 5c: Here we see a more severe penetration of the nucleus through the annulus with a greater intrusion into the spinal canal. This is also a bulging disc, or it can be called a herniated or ruptured disc.

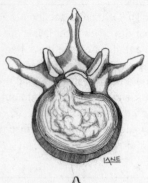

Figure 5d: Here we see a penetration of the nucleus pulposis all the way through the fibers of the annulus. This is a true ruptured disc. There is significant narrowing of the spinal canal, and major pressure against a nerve is typical.

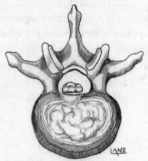

Figure 5e: Here we see a piece of ruptured disc material inside the spinal canal that is no longer attached to the disc. This is called a sequestered disc and can move up or down in the spinal canal.

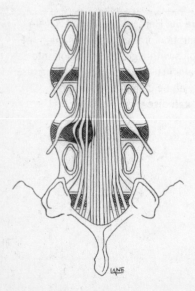

Figure 5f: This shows how a ruptured disc can press on one or more nerves, causing leg pain and perhaps weakness and numbness in the region supplied by those nerves.

Disc Degeneration

What is it?

The aging process affects every part of the body including the spine. The disc is the part of the spine that undergoes some of the most significant changes with advancing age. These changes are called disc degeneration.

Figure 6: These drawings show a degenerated disc. The upper drawing shows narrowing of the disc space and spur formation. The lower drawing shows a cross-section of the disc with an abnormal nucleus and spur formation.

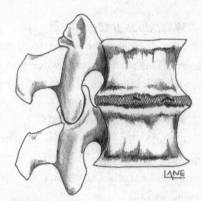

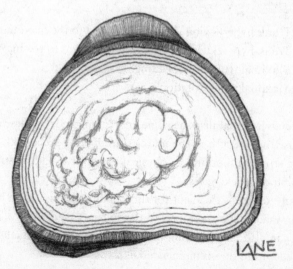

What causes it?

Beginning in early adulthood (sometimes even in the teenage years), our discs start to lose their water content and undergo other biomechanical changes that make them less flexible and less bouncy. This is a normal part of aging. Most people do not have pain with disc degeneration, but some do. It is not known exactly why. Most people see a spine doctor for disc degeneration in their 50s or 60s, but it can happen earlier or later.

What does it feel like?

Disc degeneration causes back pain but not leg pain below the knees. This pain is worse when you are sitting or standing and better when lying down. There is no weakness in the leg muscles.

How might it be treated?

Once a diagnosis of disc degeneration is made, a nonsurgical program is advised. This program recommends that you avoid positions and exercises that place stress on the painful disc. Positions to avoid include

- Trunk hyperflexion (bending forward to the maximum)
- Trunk hyperextension (bending backward to the maximum)
- Maximal trunk side-bending
- Maximal trunk rotation

Exercises to stabilize the spine are recommended. These exercises increase the strength in the muscles around the spine without mandating stressful motions. A physical therapist usually instructs you in stabilization exercises.

Pool exercise is excellent for this condition because the buoyancy of the water minimizes stress to the spine. A vigorous walking program can also be beneficial. Simple over-the-counter analgesics can be used within the recommended dosages.

If an appropriate exercise program is not beneficial, the temporary (a few weeks to months) use of a brace may help. A brace reduces pain by limiting motion. It can also cause muscle weakness, so active exercises should be continued.

Surgery is recommended only if nonsurgical approaches fail to bring pain relief. Most often, a fusion operation is performed. This involves removing the "sick" disc and filling the empty space with bone graft. In addition, the vertebrae are immobilized with screws and two small rods. Very good but not complete relief of pain is expected with this operation, since usually there is some degeneration in other discs as well.

Recently, the development of artificial discs has been in the news. At the time of this writing, artificial discs are being evaluated by the Food and Drug Administration (FDA). As of October 2004, only one type of disc has been released for general use and only for very specific situations.

Spinal Stenosis

What is it?

Spinal stenosis is a condition in which either the spinal nerves or the spinal cord become pinched because of degenerative changes in the spine. Pinching in the spinal canal is called central stenosis; pinching at the foramen is called foraminal stenosis.

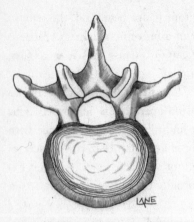

Figure 7a: This is a cross-section of a normal lumbar vertebra showing the central spinal canal including the two pedicles on either side of the spinal canal that connect the body of the vertebra (the round part) with the lamina (the roof over the spinal canal).

Figure 7b: This is the same view, but it shows loss of the normal spinal canal space due to encroachment by spurs and ligament enlargement. This condition is called spinal stenosis.

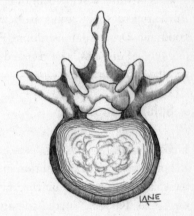

What causes it?

The aging process causes degenerative changes in the spine that can lead to spinal stenosis. For example, a degenerated disc can collapse and bulge into the spinal canal. In addition, the facet joints can become arthritic, enlarging as bone spurs develop. The net effect of these changes is diminished space in the spinal canal and/or a decrease in the foraminae (the openings where the nerves exit the spine). As these important openings narrow, the spinal cord or spinal nerves become pinched.

What does it feel like?

People with spinal stenosis often have numbness in the feet and legs. They might also have weakness in the leg and foot muscles. These symptoms are usually worse with walking and better when sitting or especially lying down. Bending forward slightly relieves the pressure on the nerves, so you will walk better leaning forward on a shopping cart than you will upright. You will also have back pain from significant disc degeneration.

How might it be treated?

This problem is usually treated two ways. First, epidural steroid injections may be tried. These are usually performed by a radiologist who injects a cortisone-type medication into the spinal canal. The goal is to reduce inflammation. Up to six injections can be done.

Surgery is the second treatment option. Surgery for central stenosis involves opening the spinal canal to allow room for the nerves. This procedure is called laminectomy and nerve root decompression. It can be done on one, two, or more levels, depending on the degree of involvement. A great improvement in leg pain, weakness, and numbness is the usual result. Sometimes back pain improves, too, but not typically since the back pain is often due to disc degeneration, which is not being treated. With more people reaching their 60s, 70s, and 80s, this operation is becoming more common.

Surgery for foraminal stenosis consists of removing the bone spurs that are compromising the foraminal opening and causing nerve compression. This surgery is called laminectomy with foraminotomy.

Degenerative Spondylolisthesis

What is it?

As our discs degenerate with age, a situation is created where one vertebra can slip forward relative to another. This slipping is called spondylolisthesis (*spondylo* means "spine" and *listhesis* means "slipping").

What causes it?

Two factors cause spondylolisthesis. As mentioned, the first factor is disc degeneration. The second factor is failed stability in the facet joints. Again, degenerative changes are the cause. The joints become arthritic and fill with fluid. This causes the stabilizing ligaments to stretch, leading to the loss of joint stability.

What does it feel like?

The main symptom with this condition is back pain. If spinal stenosis occurs with it, you may have leg pain with or without leg and foot numbness.

How might it be treated?

If your symptoms are mild, no specific treatment is needed other than following a basic back program of stabilization exercises. Stretching exercises for the back should be avoided as the spine is already too "loose."

Because looseness is the problem, your doctor may order a stabilizing brace. The brace may be worn all day or only during activities that increase your back pain. This treatment is temporary to help you through an acute episode of pain. The stabilizing exercises should be continued while you are in the brace. Epidural steroid injections may be ordered if the slipping is associated with leg pain; that is, the slipping has created spinal stenosis.

The surgical solution for spondylolisthesis is fusion. If only a one-level fusion is needed, you won't feel any stiffness since the other joints are working well. If more levels need to be fused, you are more likely to feel some stiffness. The decision on how many levels to fuse is based not just on routine X-rays but on extensive testing, possibly including MRI, discogram, CT scan, or CT myelo-gram (see Chapter 11).

Unfortunately, spondylolisthesis is often accompanied by spinal stenosis. In this case, your leg pain may be worse than your back pain. The surgical solution is a fusion (for the spondylolisthesis) and decompression (for the spinal stenosis).

Surgery for degenerative spondylolisthesis has a very high success rate. Most patients do very well and are out of the hospital in four to five days, walking on their own and taking little medication.

Osteoporosis-Related Spine Fractures

What is it?

Our bones are living structures. Throughout our lives, bone tis-sue is constantly lost and replaced. Osteoporosis is a bone disorder in which bone is lost faster than it is replaced, creating weak bones. Fractures of the hip, wrist, and especially the spine are common. Osteoporosis is more prevalent in women, especially after menopause. Osteoporosis alone does not cause back pain. Back pain is only caused by osteoporosis if a fracture occurs.

What causes it?

If you have osteoporosis, spine fractures can occur whenever there is trauma to the spine—even minor trauma such as a fall on the buttocks. Sometimes lifting something heavy or even coughing can cause a spine fracture. These are called fragility fractures.

What does it feel like?

An osteoporosis-related spine fracture can cause mild pain—so mild that you think it is just a sprain and never see a doctor. Some-times, however, the pain is more severe and requires medical care.

How might it be treated?

Treatment for this condition typically consists of pain medication and a temporary brace. Prolonged bed rest should be avoided, since more than two or three days of lying in bed will quickly cause further bone loss. A walking program should be started as soon as possible.

Surgery is very rarely required. It is only done when bone fragments crumple into the spinal canal and press on the spinal cord or spinal nerves, creating a potential for paralysis.

Recently, two procedures have been developed to treat painful osteoporosis-related compression fractures in the spine (fractures where the vertebra collapses). One procedure is vertebroplasty, which involves using a needle to inject bone cement (or a similar substance) into the fracture area, creating instant "stability." The usual result is good pain relief.

The second procedure, called kyphoplasty, is very similar. First, a balloon is placed (via needle) into the collapsed vertebra. Then the balloon is inflated, restoring the height of the vertebra. Finally, the vertebra is filled with bone cement. Complications are rare with these two procedures, but they can occur and can be quite serious, the worst being paraplegia.

No cure is available for osteoporosis, so prevention is vital. Adequate calcium and vitamin D intake along with appropriate exercise can help prevent this debilitating condition. Smoking is a big contributor to osteoporosis, especially in women.

Bone density is easily tested and medications can be prescribed if bone density is low. These medications prevent further loss, but they do not cure the condition. As of yet, there is no magic medicine to quickly make weak bones strong.

Isthmic Spondylolysis and Spondylolisthesis

What it it?

Isthmic spondylolysis is a condition in which bone is absent in a critical area of the spine (*spondylo* means "spine" and *lysis* means "absence of bone"). While the body is developing, this defect occurs in the narrow piece of bone between the facet and the laminae (the isthmus of the vertebra). The absence of bone in the isthmus may in itself produce pain. It may also cause a loss of stability in which one vertebra slips forward on the one below it. This is called spondylolisthesis (as defined previously). This slipping may be mild, moderate, or severe.

What causes it?

Spondylolysis is not present at birth, but it develops between 5 and 10 years of age. It occurs in about 5% of the population and frequently runs in families. It is more common in certain athletes, especially gymnasts.

What does it feel like?

Though typically not painful, spondylolysis causes pain in some people, especially competitive athletes. If the spondylolysis causes slipping (spondylolisthesis), then pain, numbness, and weakness may be present in the legs.

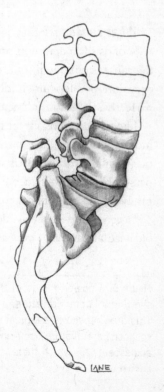

Figure 8: Here we see a lateral view of the lumbar spine with the last lumbar vertebra slipping forward on the sacrum. This isthmic spondylolisthesis is due to a defect in the posterior arch.

How might it be treated?

Treatment for isthmic spondylolisthesis depends on the severity of slippage and the severity of symptoms. For mild slips with mild symptoms, a nonsurgical program of back stabilization exercises is used. If slippage is advanced with severe pain and significant nerve pinching, then surgery is done. The vertebrae are fused, and if the nerves are pinched, decompression is also performed.

Scoliosis

What is it?

Scoliosis is a curvature of the spine from side to side, usually with rotation of the vertebrae.

What causes it?

Scoliosis is a common problem with many causes. In most cases, the cause is unknown. This is called idiopathic scoliosis. In this case, curvature develops in childhood or adolescence in a spine that was perfectly straight in infancy.

Idiopathic scoliosis is far more common in females and has a strong genetic (familial) pattern. It is commonly passed from mother to daughter but rarely passed from father to son.

Degenerative scoliosis develops in older adults and is a curvature of the

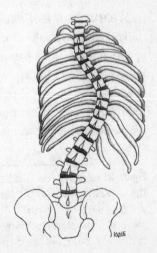

Figure 9: A posterior view of the spine showing a lateral curvature, a scoliosis. This drawing shows a typical idiopathic scoliosis, a curvature occurring in adolescents for which there is no known cause.

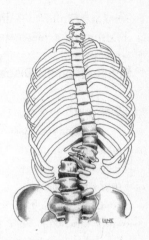

Figure 10: Another spine with scoliosis, in this case a degenerative scoliosis due to disc degeneration in an adult.

spine caused by disc and facet joint degeneration. These are milder curves than idiopathic scoliosis, but they are usually more painful.

Congenital scoliosis is caused by defects in the vertebrae that occur long before the child is born. Even though it is congenital (that is, you are born with it), it is rarely inherited from your parents. Congenital scoliosis is far less common than idiopathic scoliosis.

What does it feel like?

Adolescents with idiopathic scoliosis may or may not have mild backache, but they are able to carry on with normal life. In adulthood, however, the aching can get worse because the curvature causes degeneration in the disc and facet joints. Muscle fatigue also occurs.

How might it be treated?

Adults with scoliosis are treated in several different ways:

- Some are merely observed to see if their curves worsen. This means a yearly doctor visit and X-ray.
- If the curve steadily gets worse, fusion surgery is done.
- If the curve is bad enough to cause lung problems, correction and fusion are done.
- If the curve is small but very painful, bracing is done.
- If the curve is very painful and exercises and bracing don't help, fusion surgery is done.

Treatment in children is different. See Chapter 23 for the treatment in children and adolescents.

Scheuermann's Disease

What is it?

Scheuermann's disease causes an abnormal increase in the normal posterior curvature (kyphosis) in the mid- and upper back.

What causes it?

The cause of Scheuermann's disease is unknown. It begins in childhood and can range from very mild to very severe. It occurs equally in boys and girls and has a strong hereditary component.

What does it feel like?

Some adults with Scheuermann's disease can have an increased kyphosis but no pain. In other cases, significant pain accompanies this structural defect.

How might it be treated?

Nonsurgical treatment in adults includes pain medications and physical therapy. Physical therapy typically focuses on strengthening the extensor muscles, postural exercises, and trunk stretching into extension. This is done for pain management; there is no scientific evidence that physical therapy is effective for deformity control. See Chapter 23 for the treatment of adolescents.

Surgery may be necessary if pain is severe and there is no response to nonsurgical treatment. The operation usually involves going into the front and back of the spine to release ligaments, remove discs, and then add bone graft and instrumentation. A rare indication for this surgery is if the deformity gets so bad that it squeezes the lungs and makes breathing difficult. Lung function tests are used to assess this situation.

Less Common Back Problems

Synovial Facet Joint Cyst

This is an uncommon problem in which a cyst develops from a degenerating facet joint. This condition can cause leg pain similar to a disc herniation. The customary treatment is surgical removal of the cyst through a laminectomy.

Rheumatoid Arthritis

Rheumatoid arthritis is a severe medical problem involving inflammation of many joints. The mid- and lower back are seldom involved, but the neck is frequently problematic.

A rheumatologist manages rheumatoid arthritis–related back pain with various medications. Spine surgery is seldom needed, unless instability of the vertebrae puts the spinal cord at risk.

Ankylosing Spondylitis

Like rheumatoid arthritis, this condition involves joint inflammation, but with ankylosing spondylitis, the spine and sacroiliac joints (the joint between the sacrum and the pelvis) are often affected. As it advances, this disease can cause a bent-forward posture, sometimes so bad that you can only see the ground in front of you. Typically, ankylosing spondylitis is managed by a rheumatologist with antiinflammatory medications. If there is very poor spinal alignment, surgery can be done. However, it is very complex and should be done only by the few surgeons with adequate experience.

Infection

Spine infections are very serious. They are almost always caused by bacteria or other organisms that travel to your spine via the bloodstream from some other place in the body. Spine infections are most common in patients with diabetes or those with depressed immune systems (such as HIV or those taking cortisone or chemotherapy).

Spine infections cause mild to incredibly severe back pain. There is usually a fever, which can also range from mild to severe. Early on, routine X-rays are normal. (They change later.) An MRI will show the infection earlier. A bone scan is a very useful test, as are several lab tests.

Treatment depends on what organism or "bug" is causing the infection. Blood cultures will sometimes show what bug is involved, and an effective antibiotic is selected. Often, it is necessary to do a needle biopsy of the infected area in order to identify the bug. The antibiotic treatment is intense, starting with high-dose intravenous (IV) treatment and progressing to pills.

Surgery is indicated if an abscess is present in the spine, if there is an epidural abscess, or if the infection destroys one or more vertebral bodies.

Cancer

This is a rare cause of back pain. Metastatic cancer, which comes to the spine from somewhere else, is more common than primary cancer, which starts in the spine. Metastatic spine cancer most often comes from the breasts, lungs, prostate, or kidneys, but almost any kind of cancer can go to the spine.

The treatment for metastatic cancer usually involves radiation and/or chemotherapy. Surgery is occasionally necessary if the cancer is causing pressure on the spinal cord with resultant paralysis.

Psychological Causes of Back Pain

Some doctors, such as John Sarno, MD, of New York, feel that most back problems are caused by psychological disturbance. Sarno believes that mental tension, especially repressed anxiety, causes muscle tension. This muscle tension then causes back pain.

In reality, the causes of back pain can be put on a spectrum. On one end are those patients whose back pain is 98% psychological and 2% physical. These patients need psychotherapy rather than medication, physical therapy, or surgery.

At the other end of the spectrum are those whose back pain is 98% physical and 2% psychological. The psychological problem is usually depression caused by the back pain. Psychotherapy will not help these patients with their back pain.

Between these two extremes are situations that might be 70% physical and 30% psychological or 50% physical and 50% psychological. Proper treatment depends on proper diagnosis, so it falls upon the evaluating doctor to find the proper origin of pain and prescribe proper treatment.

There is no simple test to quickly sort out how much of a person's pain is psychological or physical. Most experts agree that doctors with good training and a lot of experience are best at arriving at a correct diagnosis.

Nonspine Causes of Pain

In this book, we strongly advocate seeing your primary care doctor early on. He or she will screen out serious problems that need immediate attention. Your doctor will also rule out nonspine causes of back pain such as kidney stones (most common), other kidney problems, enlargement of the aorta, bladder problems, or, in females, gynecological problems.

3

Nonsurgical Treatments

The treatment choices available to you as a consumer with back pain are amazing in both number and diversity. Figuring out what to do for your back can be bewildering. Will vitamins help? Do I need a new bed? Should I see a medical doctor or a chiropractor? Does acupuncture work? What about yoga?

One of the primary goals of this book is to carve a clear path for you through this tangle of treatment options. The bottom line is this: the treatment options available to you are not all equal. Some treatment choices distinguish themselves by being:

- Proven effective
- Safer to use
- Scientifically tested

Treatment choices that satisfy these valuable criteria fall under the umbrella of evidence-based medicine. To understand the relevance of evidence-based medicine in deciding how to care for your back, you must first understand the placebo effect and the body's natural healing abilities.

∎ The Placebo Effect

If a group of people with back pain is given a bottle of pills and told by the doctor to take one pill three times per day for pain relief, 30% to 40% of them will get good pain relief *even though the bottle contains only sugar pills!* Sugar pills have absolutely no ability to relieve back pain. The 30% to 40% who will get better will do so because they *believe* they will get better. This is known as the placebo effect. It attests to the power of the mind over the body. If the mind believes a certain treatment will help, 30% to 40% of the time it will, not because the treatment is effective, but because the mind convinces the body that it will work.

The placebo effect applies to all forms of back treatment, not just pills. Herbs, massage, magnets, new beds, acupuncture, and so forth—all these treatments will help 30% to 40% of the people who try them simply because their minds tell them so. To prove a certain back treatment *really* works, the placebo effect must be taken into account. The treatment must help significantly more people than the 30% to 40% who will be helped just because they are trying a new treatment. Evidence-based medicine does that. It uses and endorses back treatment options that have been shown to help more people than a placebo.

For example, if a new medicine is claimed by the drug company to be wonderful for treating back pain, those claims must be substantiated with a research study. Thousands of patients with typical back pain will be given a similar-looking pill. Unbeknownst to the patients, some will get a sugar pill while others will get the new drug. The question is: How many people will get better? If the same number of people get better with a sugar pill as with the new drug, the new drug does not really work, and it is certainly not wonderful. But if 90% of the people taking the new drug get better and only 30% of the sugar pill takers get better, we can conclude that indeed the new drug does work effectively in treating back pain.

■ The Body's Natural Healing Abilities

Along with the placebo effect, evidence-based medicine takes into account the power of the body's natural healing ability. All of us have witnessed this power. We have seen paper cuts heal and scraped knees get better. Maybe you broke a bone once and today it is as good as new.

Most people with back pain get better because of the natural healing power of their own body. Your simplest (and cheapest) healing ally is the ability of the body to heal itself.

Evidence-based medicine doesn't use or endorse a treatment unless it helps your body heal better than it would on its own. How is that proven? A research project is designed in which one group of patients with back pain gets a new kind of treatment while another group gets nothing at all. Again, the question is: How many people get better? If the same number of patients gets better in both groups, then the new treatment is no better than the body's ability to heal itself. But if a significant number of people get better with the new treatment in comparison to those who did not get the treatment, the new treatment has been shown to work better than the body's ability to heal itself.

■ The Solid Ground of Evidence-Based Medicine

If Aunt Matilda tells you that she wore a copper bracelet and her back pain went away, there is no way to tell if she experienced the placebo effect (she got better because she believed she would) or if the body's natural healing ability was at work (she would have gotten better even if she had not tried the bracelet). Many types of back treatment options have no evidence to prove they are any better than a placebo or the body's natural healing ability. Evidence-based medicine uses research to prove that a medication or treatment option is more than a placebo and better than your body's own healing ability.

As we discuss back treatment choices in this book, we will clearly delineate which treatments have solid evidence to support their use, which have some evidence to support their use, and which have none at all. Choosing the treatment(s) that is supported by solid evidence gives you the best chance of safely getting better faster. It is, of course, okay to try any treatment approach you want as long as you understand that once you step off the path of evidence-based medicine, you are on less solid ground.

▌Self-Care

Self-care is the best way to begin effectively treating your back. It is simply those things that you do for yourself to enhance your recovery.

Self-care starts with a commitment to get up and get moving. Over time, you may have developed a protective attitude toward your back. But people who give in to the pain and stop moving do not get well. Walking is a safe and excellent way to stay in shape (or get back in shape) while your back heals. If you have been given an exercise program by a doctor or physical therapist, do it. In the short run, it helps your acute pain. In the long run, it builds a stronger back.

If you are overweight, losing weight can really help your back. Extra weight means extra load and stress on the back. Your family doctor can help direct you to a safe and effective weight-loss program.

If you smoke, it's time to quit. There is no question that smoking hinders healing. Ask your family doctor to help you find a program to stop smoking.

Avoid overloading your spine. Do not lift heavy objects, sit for prolonged periods, or do repetitive bending and twisting. Eventually, you will get back to doing those things, but right now your back needs a chance to heal.

Taking over-the-counter medications such as aspirin, Tylenol (acetaminophen), or Advil and Motrin (ibuprofen) is okay in recommended doses. Avoid calling your doctor for narcotic medications. They can make you sick and run a high risk for addiction.

Remember to care for emotions as well. Work to adopt a positive outlook. Be hopeful, too. After all, caring for your back and your emotions is a great step toward getting better.

▌ Medications

Before becoming available to consumers and patients, medications must undergo strenuous testing for safety and effectiveness. The process is not foolproof—there are still some medications that get through testing and later prove to be harmful—but in general this testing procedure helps ensure a medication is safe and effective.

Medications can be a great help to those with back pain if the correct medicine is given at the correct dosage for the correct period of time. The benefits of any medication must be balanced against its general side effects. Your personal allergy history must be considered before a medication is prescribed, as well as the potential for the medication to conflict with any others you might be using. Remember, pain medications never treat the cause of the pain; they merely cover it up while your natural healing abilities treat the cause.

Over-the-Counter Medications

These medications are readily available to anyone with back pain. They can be used for acute, subacute, or chronic pain. The dosage on the label should always be followed. Each of these medications may cause certain complications depending on your own medical problems, how many you take per day, and for how long.

Pain Medication

Tylenol (acetaminophen) is a common pain medication. In contrast to aspirin, it does not have any antiinflammatory qualities, and it does not have a tendency to cause bleeding. Consequently, it is a good pain medicine to use if you are going to have surgery. Follow the recommended dosage. If taken in excess, acetaminophen can cause liver problems.

Pain and Antiinflammatory Medications

Aspirin is a well-known pain medication with some antiinflammatory qualities. When taken in its usual dose, it is quite safe. Because it can interfere with blood clotting, it should not be taken by people with stomach ulcers or other bleeding problems. In some people, aspirin irritates the stomach. Enteric-coated aspirin is easier on the stomach. Aspirin should not be taken before surgery, since it may increase bleeding during surgery. If you are scheduled for surgery, ask your doctor how long before surgery you should avoid aspirin.

Advil and Motrin (ibuprofen) are pain and antiinflammatory medications. They are chemically different from aspirin and Tylenol (acetaminophen). The antiinflammatory abilities of ibuprofen qualify this medication as a nonsteroidal antiinflammatory drug (NSAID). Like aspirin and all of the NSAIDs, ibuprofen can cause bleeding and should not be taken prior to surgery.

Alleve and Naprosyn (naproxen) are NSAIDs. They are similar to ibuprofen, but chemically they are slightly different. They can also cause bleeding and should not be taken before surgery.

Cartilage-Enhancing Medications for Arthritis or Joint Degeneration

Glucosamine is used for degenerative arthritis of the joints. Because glucosamine is an important component of cartilage, it is thought this medication can help restore damaged joints including the facet joints of the spine. There is no scientific evidence that it has benefit for back pain.

Chondroitin sulfate is also found in cartilage and is usually taken with glucosamine to treat joint arthritis or degeneration. There is no scientific evidence as yet that it has value for back pain.

Prescription Medications

Prescription medications are prescribed for you by a physician who knows your present condition and your health history. Always use prescription medications according to the instructions given by your doctor.

Muscle Relaxants

Muscle relaxants are prescribed for acute muscle spasms. They have been shown to have some benefit for acute back pain, but their use does not decrease disability.

Robaxin (methocarbamol) is a commonly prescribed muscle relaxant. It is most helpful for acute muscles spasms and has no benefit for chronic back problems.

Flexeril (cyclobenzaprine) is a commonly prescribed muscle relaxant.

Soma (carisoprodol) is a commonly prescribed muscle relaxant.

Pain Medications

Prescription pain medications range from moderate pain relief (with moderate potential for addiction) to heavy pain relief (with heavy potential for addiction). For this reason, these medications are carefully prescribed by doctors and closely controlled by the Drug Enforcement Administration (DEA). If you take these medications, always carefully follow the prescribed dosage and do not prolong their use. Remember, pain medications do not fix your problem. They only decrease your pain while your body's natural healing abilities work.

Codeine is probably the most commonly used pain medication. It can be prescribed in its pure form, but it is often combined with other medications. Tylenol #3 is 30 mg of codeine combined with 300 mg of Tylenol. Tylenol #4 is 60 mg of codeine combined with 300 mg of Tylenol.

Darvon (propoxyphene) is a prescription pain medicine often combined with other nonprescription medications such as Darvon Compound (Darvon plus aspirin and caffeine) or Darvocet (Darvon plus acetaminophen).

Ultram (tramadol) is yet another prescription pain medication for moderate to moderately severe pain. It is said to have fewer sedative effects than other narcotics.

Vicodin (hydrocodone) is a commonly used narcotic medication for moderate to moderately severe pain. It is often used as a "going-home" oral pain medication after surgery. Vicodin ES and Narco are Vicodin plus acetaminophen, and Vicoprophen is Vicodin plus ibuprofen.

Percodan (oxycodone) is prescribed for moderate to moderately severe pain. It is quite addictive if taken for too long a period of time. Percocet (oxycodone and acetaminophen) is, of course, very similar to Percodan. Tylot is essentially the same thing, but it is made by a different company.

Demerol (meperidine) is a prescription medication for moderately severe to severe pain. It can be highly addictive.

Dilaudid (hydromorphone) is a prescription medication for moderately severe to severe pain. Like Demerol, it is highly addictive.

Oxycontin (oxycodone) is prescribed for moderately severe to severe pain. It has, unfortunately, become overprescribed and is highly addictive. It has also become a popular street drug. (We are currently in an epidemic of people addicted to this medication.)

Morphine is used only for severe pain, usually for a few days after surgery. It is highly addictive. It is also used in morphine pumps (see Chapter 4).

Duragesic (fentanyl patch) is prescribed for chronic pain not responsive to lesser analgesics. Like narcotics, it can be addictive.

Neurontin (gabapentin) is a nonnarcotic analgesic used for epileptic seizures and for the pain of shingles. It is sometimes prescribed for patients with chronic nerve pain in the leg.

Tegretol (carbamazepine) and Dilantin (phenytoin) are medications also used primarily for epileptic seizures. Like Neurontin, they are occasionally prescribed for nerve pain.

Three NSAIDs deserve special mention: Vioxx, Bextra, and Celebrex. They are called Cox-2 inhibitors, since they have a different chemical background than the other NSAIDs such as Advil, Aleve, Naprosyn, and so on. Both Vioxx and Bextra have been removed from the market by the FDA because they have been linked to an increased risk of heart attacks and strokes. As of the writing of this book, Celebrex has not been removed from the market, but advertising has been stopped and stronger warnings have been placed on the bottles.

Physical Therapy

Physical therapy is a tried-and-true method for treating back pain. Though often viewed as just exercise or massage, physical therapy is actually a highly individualized treatment package of various techniques prescribed and applied by a professional after a thorough evaluation.

A physical therapist might use several modalities (types of treatment) to treat your back pain including ice, heat, massage, stretching, ultrasound, posture training, body mechanics instruction, and manual techniques. Physical therapists use many different types of exercise including active flexion, active extension, active lateral bending, active torsion (oblique strengthening), spine stabilization, isometrics, and exercise ball programs.

Your specific physical therapy program will depend on your doctor's recommendation and the physical therapy evaluation. Sometimes physical therapy involves a bit of trial and error to find the approach that is best for you.

You will find a thorough overview of physical therapy in Chapter 15. A summary of the evidence to support physical therapy in the treatment of back pain is also included. Research indicates that physical therapy is particularly helpful in treating subacute and chronic back pain. Physical therapy is considered part of the conventional medical system and is almost always covered by insurance.

Chiropractic

The role of chiropractic in the care of spine problems has long been controversial. Even today, chiropractors are seen as skilled spine doctors by some and total quacks by others. In reality, there is some evidence to support the use of chiropractic care for back pain in specific situations.

Chiropractors are graduates of schools of chiropractic where they receive two to four years of training. They are not required to have a college degree and they are not graduates of medical school (though they call themselves "doctor"). They are identified by the letters DC (doctor of chiropractic).

Traditionally, chiropractors have attributed back pain to "subluxations," or a partial displacement of the facet joints in the back. The common terminology is having your back "out" or "out of alignment." Chiropractors treat subluxations with manipulation or a specifically directed thrust applied sharply to the back to "relocate" the subluxed vertebrae or "realign" the back.

There is no scientific evidence that subluxations actually exist. Often, patients have X-rays taken and they are told that the X-rays show subluxations, but they don't really exist. Perhaps a more likely explanation is that muscle spasms in the short muscles of the spine cause acute back pain, and chiropractic manipulation stretches these muscles, which brings pain relief.

The scientific evidence supporting chiropractic care was summarized in the *Journal of the American Academy of Orthopedic Surgery* in 2003. The article states that chiropractic is often as good as other approaches for treating acute back pain. Chiropractic is not as effective for subacute back pain and generally not effective for chronic back conditions. If your family doctor has ruled out cancer, infection, osteoporosis, and referral of pain to the spine from outside the spine and you want to try chiropractic, it is probably all right. If chiropractic care is going to work for you, you will begin to feel relief in just a few sessions. A good chiropractor will

- Discharge you promptly once you reach maximum improvement or if you are not better after a few sessions
- Not ask you to sign a contract or recommend "maintenance" adjustments
- Provide you with rehabilitation exercises and active care such as a home program
- Not be "subluxation" focused, since this idea has no scientific evidence

Be sure to check with your insurance to company to see if chiropractic care is covered in your policy.

Epidural Steriod Injections

This procedure involves the injection of steroid medications into the epidural space (the space outside the dural sac but inside the spinal canal). It is an invasive technique, meaning the medication is actually placed inside the body, but it is not considered surgery.

The steroid injection is usually done by a radiologist under X-ray guidance. The steroid medication is a strong cortisone-like antiin-flammatory medication. It stays in the injected area—it does not spread throughout the body—which allows it to have a strong local effect.

This procedure is used to treat the irritated nerves in spinal stenosis (see Chapter 2). Up to six treatments can be administered with the goal of reducing back and especially leg symptoms. Epidural steroid injections are often used to prevent or at least delay surgery. This procedure typically yields a very positive benefit.

Nerve Root Blocks

Nerve root blocks are used both to treat and diagnose back problems when nerve pain is present from one specific nerve. Under X-ray guidance, a doctor (usually a radiologist) places a needle into the space where the nerve comes out of the spine (but not into the nerve) and a local anesthetic is injected. The anesthetic numbs the nerve. If the pain goes away, the doctor knows exactly what nerve is involved. Then, the radiologist will inject some steroid (antiinflam-matory) medicine into the same area. The local anesthetic wears off in an hour or two, but the steroid injection lasts longer. This invasive, nonsurgical procedure is similar to epidural steroid injection for spinal stenosis.

A recent study was done on a group of patients with disc herniation causing severe nerve pain into the leg. Surgery was planned for each of these patients. They received a nerve root block, and many had such good relief that their surgery was canceled.

Massage

Massage is a touch therapy using certain strokes and techniques to manipulate soft tissue (skin, muscles, tendons). There are many schools of massage. They are often classified by whether they apply light, moderate, or deep touch. Traditional or Swedish massage uses gliding strokes, kneading, friction, and tapping with a moderately vigorous touch.

Rolfing is a massage technique that uses very deep touch. Rolfing typically involves a ten-session series, each building on the previous one. Another type of massage is called myofascial release (*myo* means "muscle" and *fascia* is the fibrous tissue around the muscle). The theory behind this treatment technique is that tight muscles and fascia cause back pain (or contribute to movement dysfunctions that eventually lead to back problems). In reality, there is no proof that myofascial tightness exists. Myofascial release is really just another form of deep massage.

In the United States, massage is considered a complementary or alternative treatment, whereas in Europe it is considered conventional medicine for back pain. In Austria, for example, 87% of patients with back pain receive (and are reimbursed for) massage.

A look at the overall evidence to support massage as a treatment for back pain is encouraging but not compelling. Evidence supports the use of massage for acute lower back pain, but its value is considered limited for chronic lower back pain. If you are inclined to try massage for your back problem, go ahead. The risks are very low and it might very well help.

Ask your doctor, physical therapist, or chiropractor for a referral to a good massage therapist. There are many ways to become a massage therapist, some requiring much more education and training than others. One of the most reputable organizations is the American Medical Massage Association (AMMA). Members of this organization are required to graduate from a school licensed by the State Department of Education and to complete six hundred hours of supervised training with significant emphasis on neurological and musculoskeletal pathology. Use the yellow pages in the phone book or the AMMA website to find a medical massage therapist (www.americanmedicalmassage.com). Unless it is performed by a physical therapist as part of your physical therapy program, massage is usually not covered by insurance in the United States.

Pilates

Pilates is an exercise program that emphasizes strengthening of the core body muscles—the trunk, back, abdominal, pelvis, and thigh muscles. These muscles are important for a healthy back. In addition, posture and breathing awareness are part of this program. Some Pilates exercises can be done on the floor or an exercise mat, whereas others require special equipment. Pilates is more vigorous than most back exercises, so it is not recommended for acute back pain. It can be good for maintaining a healthy back if you start slowly, gradually increase the program intensity, and can perform the exercises without aggravating your back pain. There is no solid evidence to support the use of Pilates exercises as a specific intervention for back pain, although strengthening exercises in general can be helpful.

Many physical therapists have some training in Pilates exercises, and that might be the safest way for you to get started. Training for Pilates instructors ranges from a weekend of training to several hundred hours. If you take a Pilates class, ask the instructor about his or her training background. In general, those with more training are better prepared to teach this program. If you want to try a videotape, Stott Pilates videos are considered reputable. They can be found in sporting good stores or on the Internet (www.stottpilates.com).

Yoga

Yoga was developed approximately five thousand years ago in India, so it has a long history of practice. It combines physical postures or positions with breathing (some methods also include meditation). There are literally dozens of different types of yoga, but the most widely used method is Hatha yoga. This method uses a series of body movements and positions that involve stretching and holding, as well as breathing exercises. Holding positions requires muscle use, which helps the muscles become stronger. The stretching component can also be beneficial for those with back pain. In summary, the practice of yoga is consistent with recommendations for back pain patients to be active. There is very little scientific evidence that yoga actually helps back patients, but it will likely improve your flexibility, balance, and strength, which should be beneficial.

Yoga classes are often offered at health clubs, the local YMCA, and yoga studios. You can also look up yoga in the yellow pages. If you prefer a yoga videotape, Yogafit (www.yogafit.com) is one of the most respected names in the field. You can find Yogafit's videotapes in sporting good stores or on the Internet.

Vitamins

Vitamins are good for your general health but have no specific value in alleviating back pain. Vitamin D plays a role in spinal health because it helps the body absorb calcium, which is important in bone metabolism and in preventing osteoporosis.

Braces

Braces have been used for centuries and continue to be useful in certain situations. Braces work by limiting movements so that the back can heal. They are used for symptom management, not to treat the cause of the back pain. Situations where braces are helpful are those where the vertebrae are truly unstable such as with spondylolisthesis. If stabilizing exercises aren't effective, a brace can be used to decrease instability. Braces are extensively used for treatment of certain spine fractures.

Adolescents with spine curvatures such as idiopathic scoliosis and Scheuermann's kyphosis might wear a brace to control the curve (not to relieve pain). In older adults with degenerative scoliosis, a brace may be used for pain relief (not to correct the curve).

These types of braces are prescribed by a spine doctor and custom made by an orthotist (brace maker). Studies have shown that "off-the-shelf" back supports or corsets are not a worthwhile treatment for back pain. You might consider temporarily (a few days) wearing one if you have an acute episode. It can limit painful movements and give a feeling of support. Long-term use is not helpful, since muscle weakness will result from disuse of muscles.

Acupuncture

Acupuncture has been around for thousands of years and has been gaining popularity in North America since the 1980s. This treatment uses fine needles to stimulate specific points in the body that represent so-called pathways for energy flow. There is no evidence to validate the theory behind acupuncture and no evidence to support its use in treating back pain.

Psychotherapy

Almost every medical doctor recognizes the influence the mind can have on back pain, but that does not mean that every back problem can be cured with psychotherapy. If your back pain is caused by psychological and emotional factors, then psychotherapy is appropriate. However, if you have a ruptured disc or disc degeneration or any physical cause for your back pain, psychotherapy is not the answer. You cannot use mental techniques to relieve pain caused by a bone spur pressing on your nerve.

In his book *The Mind–Body Connection*, Dr. John Sarno states that most back pain is due to muscle tension caused by repressed mental anxiety. The author says that in most cases the cure for back pain is psychotherapy and that any type of medical treatment such as physical therapy should not be done. Dr. Sarno makes this claim even though he is not a psychiatrist (he is a physical medicine and rehabilitation specialist).

We hold a different position. Back surgeons often see patients who have a long, frustrating history of seeking nonsurgical solutions, including psychotherapy, to their back problems without success. When they finally arrive at the spine surgeon's office, they are depressed. Once a surgical solution is found and major pain relief occurs, the depression goes away. They were depressed because they had years of daily back pain—a situation that would cause depression in many people.

Two major studies have shown that people with depression and back pain are almost always depressed because of chronic pain, and that prior to the back pain, depression wasn't an issue. In addition, treating most patients with back pain using antidepressant medications has not worked.

Special Beds

When it comes to back pain and beds, there are two things you should know:

1. A soft, sagging mattress tends to aggravate lower back pain.
2. A firm—not rock-hard—mattress is best.

All the hype about expensive special beds for back problems is unsubstantiated. Instead of wasting your money on a special bed, try changing your sleeping position. The side-lying position with hips and knees flexed tends to work best for people with back problems. If you sleep on your back, use the contour position (see Fig. 1, p. 8).

Traction

Many years ago, traction (stretching the spine by elongation) was a popular way to treat back pain. Patients with miserable backaches were admitted to the hospital for a week of constant traction in the contour position with a heating pad and pain medication. This is no longer done because it was shown to be no more effective than two to three days at home in the contour position with a heating pad and some pain medications.

Traction can also be done in the doctor's office. It can feel good while it is being applied, but the benefit rapidly disappears when you sit or stand.

Copper Bracelets

Neither your health nor your back pain will benefit from copper bracelets.

Magnets

There is no evidence to support the use of magnets for your backache or any other health problem.

TENS Units

A TENS (transcutaneous electrical nerve stimulation) unit is a small device that hooks on the waist band of your pants. It has thin wires that connect to small pads stuck to your back. Electrical impulses are transmitted from the unit into your body through the skin. The theory is that the electrical impulses will block the transmission of pain signals to your brain. There is presently no evidence to support the use of TENS in the treatment of back pain.

Massaging Recliner Chairs

These chairs can feel good while you sit in them, but they offer no lasting benefit.

Prolotherapy

This treatment involves injection of a local anesthetic or some other substance into tender areas. It can temporarily numb a painful area, but it has no long-term benefit.

IDET

Intradiscal electrothermography involves using an electric current that is passed into the disc by a long needle to "heat" the disc and "heal" tears in the annulus. There is no solid evidence that it has any value.

Facet Rhizotomy

This is another technique that attempts to treat facet joint pain by inserting needles near the joints and using radiofrequency coagulation to destroy the little nerves in the area. This treatment approach has been proven ineffective except in a few patients with pure facet joint disease.

Chemonucleolysis

This is yet another obsolete treatment approach in which an enzyme is injected into the disc. It has been proven ineffective and occasionally even life-threatening due to severe allergic reactions.

■▪■■▪■■■▪■■■▪■■▪■■■▪■■▪■■■▪■■▪■■■▪■■▪■■■▪■■▪■■■▪■■■■

SUMMARY OF EFFECTIVENESS OF NONSURGICAL TREATMENT APPROACHES FOR BACK PAIN

Most Effective Treatments
(supported by solid evidence)

Medications
(when used correctly)

Physical Therapy
(especially for subacute and chronic back problems)

Epidural Steroid Injections
(used to treat spinal stenosis)

Most Effective Treatments *(cont'd)*
(supported by solid evidence)

Nerve Root Blocks
(used to diagnose and treat nerve pain)

Chiropractic
(particularly effective with acute back pain)

Moderately Effective Treatments
(supported by some evidence)

Massage

Facet Rhizotomy

Pilates/Yoga
(The strengthening and stretching components can help with conditioning.)

Braces
(used to manage symptoms)

Least Effect Treatments
(no supportive evidence or proven ineffective)

Vitamins
(necessary for healthy living but not a specific aid in healing back problems)

Acupuncture

Special Beds

Traction

Copper Bracelets

Magnets

TENS Units

Massaging Recliner Chairs

Prolotherapy

IDET

Chemonucleolysis

Effective for Special Cases

Psychotherapy
(used when emotional or psychological factors are the main cause of back pain)

4

Surgical Treatments

The purpose of this chapter is to present and explain in under-standable language the nature of the various surgeries for problems of the spine that cause pain. Surgical procedures are presented in approximate order of frequency. If you are reading this, you have probably been told that you need surgery and you want to educate yourself as to what will be done. Chapter 2 explained the many different causes of back pain and gave some indications for when surgery is needed for certain problems. The potential risks and complications of any surgery are many, and they vary considerably from patient to patient as well as from one surgery to another. We strongly urge you to discuss these potential risks with your surgeon. Chapter 16 will help you in asking the proper questions.

■ What Are the Spine Operations?

- Decompression Operations
  - *Lumbar hemilaminotomy and disc fragment removal*
  - *Laminectomy and spinal canal decompression for spinal stenosis*

- *Anterior discectomy for thoracic disc herniation*
- *Endoscopic decompression for lumbar disc herniation*
- **Fusion Operations**
  - *Anterior lumbar interbody fusion (ALIF) with bone grafts*
  - *Anterior lumbar interbody fusion with stand-alone cage*
  - *Anterior thoracic or lumbar fusion with strut graft or cylindrical cage*
  - *Lumbar posterolateral fusion*
  - *Lumbar posterolateral fusion with instrumentation*
  - *Posterior lumbar interbody fusion (PLIF)*
  - *Transforaminal lumbar interbody fusion (TLIF)*
  - *Posterior instrumentation and fusion for spinal deformity*
  - *Combined anterior interbody fusion and posterolateral fusion with instrumentation*
  - *Posterior fusion mass osteotomy and refusion*
  - *Pedicle subtraction osteotomy and refusion*
  - *Fusion with bone morphogenetic protein (BMP)*
- **Other Operations**
  - *Artificial disc replacement*
  - *Vertebroplasty*
  - *Kyphoplasty*
  - *Thoracoplasty*
  - *Pars interarticularis repair*
  - *Artificial ligaments*
  - *Interspinous spacers*
  - *Morphine pump*
  - *Spinal cord stimulation*

Decompression Operations

Decompression operations are done to relieve pressure on the spinal nerves or spinal cord. They can be either emergency (rare) or elective (common) procedures. The exact procedure depends on the specific problem.

Lumbar Hemilaminotomy and Disc Fragment Removal

A small incision is made in the lower back, and two laminae and the ligaments are exposed on one side. The yellow ligament (ligamentum flavum) is opened along with the removal of a little bit of bone. This allows the surgeon to look into the spinal canal, gently move the pinched nerve to one side, and then remove the herniated disc fragment. The entire disc is not removed, only the herniated fragment and other loose fragments that may be nearby. A microdiscectomy is the same operation done with the aid of an operating microscope or loupe magnification. The patient usually goes home the same day or the next day. No bed rest is required.

Laminectomy and Spinal Canal Decompression for Spinal Stenosis

The surgeon must first decide how many levels need decompression. This is determined before surgery through the various imaging and clinical examination tests. A midline incision is made in the back, the muscles are moved aside, and the spine is exposed. One or more laminae are removed, exposing the spinal canal and nerve roots. The surgeon then removes whatever might be compressing the nerves, such as disc material, bone spurs, and ligaments. This usually includes looking at the nerves as they go out of the foramen (foraminal decompression). The muscles that have been moved aside to do the decompression are then placed back in their normal position. Patients usually go home in two to three days. Recovery is longer than for simple discectomy, but bed rest is not required.

Anterior Discectomy for Thoracic Disc Herniation

Thoracic disc ruptures are far rarer than lumbar disc ruptures. In the lumbar spine, disc ruptures are removed through a posterior approach, but in the thoracic spine things are different. The difference is that the spinal cord is lying over the disc and a surgeon cannot

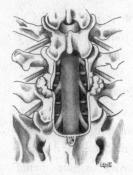

Figure 11a: This drawing shows a typical decompression operation for spinal stenosis. The laminar arches have been removed, and the nerves have been fully freed from any ligament, bone, or disc pressure.

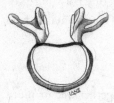

Figure 11b: A cross-section of a lumbar vertebra after a decompression for spinal stenosis.

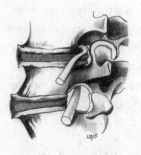

Figure 11c: A lateral view of the lumbar spine showing at the upper disc level a nerve exiting the spine through a foramen. The nerve is compressed by bone spurs and disc material. This condition is called foraminal stenosis. The lower disc level shows what has been done surgically: the opening up of the foramen by removal of whatever is pinching the nerve.

move the spinal cord to one side to remove the disc. Thus, most (but not all) thoracic disc herniations are removed through an anterior approach. The exception is a far-lateral disc, which can be removed posteriorly.

The anterior approach is through the chest, either by an open procedure in which a piece of rib is removed or by the use of a thoracoscope (a tube inserted through a small hole in the chest, which uses a video camera and special instruments to do the surgery). A typical hospital stay is three to four days.

Endoscopic Decompression for Lumbar Disc Herniation

This decompression operation is done through a narrow tube with video camera assistance. The problems with this procedure include the surgeon's limited field of vision and the likelihood that he or she will remove an inadequate amount of tissue. A fundamental rule in surgery is that if you can't get a good view of what you're doing, you can't perform a successful operation. This is usually done as an outpatient.

Fusion Operations

Fusion operations are designed to "weld" together one or more of the motion segments of the spine. This is done for a large variety of reasons including local instability, localized pain problems, fractures, and spinal deformities. These operations are discussed according to whether the front part of the spine is operated on or the posterior (back) part. Sometimes it is necessary to do both an anterior and posterior fusion. These fusions are two separate operations, but done on the same day under one anesthetic. The usual hospital stay is five to seven days.

Anterior Lumbar Interbody Fusion (ALIF) with Bone Grafts

A surgeon makes an incision in the lower abdominal area, most often to the left of the midline. The length of the incision usually depends on the number of levels to be fused. After getting down to the spine, the surgeon removes part of the annulus and then removes about 90% to 95% of the disc. Once the disc is removed, the empty space is filled with bone grafts. These can be small chips of bone or solid pieces, the choice depending on the goal to be accomplished. The bone can be either your own (autograft) or someone else's (allo-

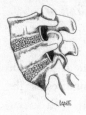

Figure 12: This side view of the lower two discs shows the disc material for removal and replacement by bone chips. This is one type of anterior interbody fusion.

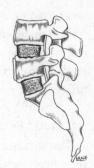

Figure 13: This side view of the lower two discs shows the disc material for removal and replacement by solid pieces of bone graft. This is another type of anterior interbody fusion.

graft), again the choice depending on various factors. This operation is almost always accompanied by a posterior fusion and fixation.

Anterior Lumbar Interbody Fusion (ALIF) with Stand-Alone Cage

In the early 1990s, the concept was promoted that the surgeon could go in the front of the spine, remove the bad disc, and screw in two hollow cylindrical cages filled with bone grafts. Thousands and thousands of these procedures were done and are still being done in some places. At the Twin Cities Spine Center, we have tried this procedure but with very disappointing results in our own patients. Also used are femoral ring allografts or square cages. We have also had quite a few patients operated on elsewhere who have been referred to us for salvage of their failed stand-alone cage surgery. As the high percent of failure has become more obvious, fewer and fewer of these procedures are now being done. A typical hospital stay is two to three days.

Anterior Thoracic or Lumbar Fusion with Strut Graft or Cylindrical Cage

This is a rarely used procedure as it is reserved for certain severe fractures, tumors, or infections. The surgeon opens the front of the spine, removes the offending vertebral body, decompresses the spinal canal, and replaces the missing vertebral body with strong ("strut") bone grafts or a metallic cylinder filled with bone. Metal implants to provide stability can be added anteriorly at the same time or done posteriorly, usually under the same anesthetic.

Lumbar Posterolateral Fusion

The surgeon exposes the back of the spine including the transverse processes through a midline incision. After cleaning the bones of all bits of muscle or other soft tissues, the bone surfaces are roughened and bone graft is added. This bone graft is usually the patient's own bone taken from the back of the pelvis, but through the same incision. A typical hospital stay is four to five days.

Lumbar Posterolateral Fusion with Instrumentation

This is the same posterolateral fusion, but with the addition of internal fixation with screws placed in the pedicles and connected to

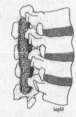

Figure 14: This shows a posterolateral fusion. The bone chips have been placed on the posterior elements of the vertebra including the transverse processes, the laminae, the facet joints, and the spinous process.

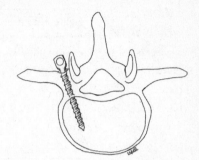

Figure 15: This cross-section of a lumbar vertebra shows a screw placed down a pedicle. Typically screws are placed in both pedicles of every vertebra included in the fusion area.

each other with little rods. The addition of internal fixation allows quicker rehabilitation and more secure bone healing. Some surgeons use translaminar screw fixation, but we have found this technique less effective.

Posterior Lumbar Interbody Fusion (PLIF)

A laminectomy is performed and the nerves are pushed to the side. The surgeon then removes the posterior annulus, removes most of the disc, and inserts bone grafts into the disc space from behind. This is usually combined with posterior fixation. The surgeons of the Twin Cities Spine Center will do this procedure only in rare circumstances, the complication rate being excessively high in our opinion, particularly scarring around the nerves. A typical hospital stay is four to five days.

Transforaminal Lumbar Interbody Fusion (TLIF)

This newer procedure allows the surgeon to do the disc removal and bone grafting through the posterior incision, and it avoids a majority of the nerve root retraction and bleeding into the spinal canal that is such a problem with the PLIF procedure. A full laminectomy is not necessary. The bones in the back are held together securely with small screws and rods, then bone graft is added. A typical hospital stay is three to four days.

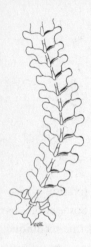

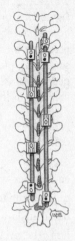

Figure 16a: A posterior view of a spine with scoliosis before correction.

Figure 16b: The same spine after correction with metallic rods and hooks. A posterior fusion is then done.

Posterior Instrumentation and Fusion for Spinal Deformity

This is the most common of the operations for the treatment of scoliosis and has been successfully used since 1960. The spine is exposed through a midline posterior incision, any tight ligaments are released, and then rods with hooks, pedicle screws, or wires, or a combination of them, are applied to the spine in such a way that the deformity is partially corrected. Bone grafts are then added and the incision is closed. The number of fused vertebrae depends on the length and complexity of the deformity. With modern fixation techniques, a cast or brace is seldom needed after the surgery. A typical hospital stay is five to seven days.

Combined Anterior Interbody Fusion and Posterolateral Fusion with Instrumentation

This is a combination of bone grafting of the disc space through an anterior approach and posterior fixation with small screws and rods. This procedure is common, with a five- to seven-day hospital stay.

Posterior Fusion Mass Osteotomy and Refusion

If you had a fracture of your femur (thigh bone) and for some reason it healed in a crooked position, the orthopedic surgeon could do an osteotomy (the cutting of bone) of the thigh bone, put it into correct alignment, and then fix it there with some type of rod or plate.

Similarly, a spine surgeon can do an osteotomy of the spine to correct a rigid deformity. The spine is, however, much more complicated than the thigh bone, since it has the spinal cord and nerves running through it.

One type of spinal osteotomy is used to treat patients who previously had a posterior spine fusion for a spinal deformity or back pain but have a persistent deformity problem. In this situation, the front of the spine has not had surgery before.

The surgeon does a posterior fusion mass osteotomy, often called a Smith-Petersen osteotomy. The surgeon reopens the old posterior incision, finds the old fusion, and takes a segment of bone out of the fusion mass. This can be done at one or multiple levels. Then the surgeon inserts some type of metal device to correct the deformity and to hold the bones still while they knit together. This procedure is often combined with an anterior discectomy and anterior interbody fusion. The hospital stay is quite variable depending on the problem.

Pedicle Subtraction Osteotomy and Refusion

A second type of osteotomy is called a pedicle subtraction osteotomy. It is used primarily in patients who have had a previous fusion and have lost their normal lumbar lordosis. It is also used in patients with ankylosing spondylitis.

The surgeon opens up the back and takes out a larger wedge of bone from the old fusion mass. He or she then removes a pair of pedicles (the reason for the name *pedicle subtraction*) and proceeds forward into the vertebral body and discs until a wedge of bone in front of the dural sac has been removed. Metal implants are then used to close the wedge, thus restoring better alignment. This complex and difficult procedure should be done only by surgeons with considerable experience. The typical hospital stay is five to seven days.

Fusion with Bone Morphogenetic Protein (BMP)

BMP is the naturally occurring substance that our bodies produce in order to heal a fracture or create a spine fusion. Scientists have learned how to create this substance artificially so that it can be used to stimulate a spine fusion. It appears to be a major advance in bone healing biology. At the time of this writing, the FDA has released BMP for extremely limited and highly regulated use in the United States. It is extremely expensive, costing about four thousand dollars for a one-level fusion, and it may or may not be covered by your insurance. It will be several years before all of the clinical research has been completed and thus the true value of BMP is determined. Hopefully, the price will have come down considerably by that time.

Other Operations

These are mostly operations that are neither decompressions nor fusions.

Artificial Disc Replacement

Artificial discs have been used for about ten years at several centers in Europe, especially France and Germany. There have been some very excellent results and some very poor results. At the present time, the FDA, the government agency responsible for new drugs and new surgical implants, has begun a series of trials in the Unites States at several centers and under very strict control. In October 2004, the FDA approved one of the designs, the Charite, for limited use. It appears from the information now available that the

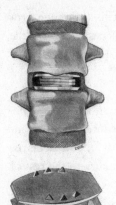

Figure 17: An artificial disc.

best results are in patients with a single level of disc degeneration, a minimal amount of disc collapse, no degeneration of the facet joints, and no osteoporosis. Relatively few people meet all of these criteria. A failed artificial disc is very difficult to fix. A typical hospital stay is two to three days.

Vertebroplasty

This procedure is done for patients with painful compression fractures due to osteoporosis (see Chapter 2). Under sedation and local anesthesia, the doctor (spine surgeon or radiologist) passes a large needle down a pedicle into the fractured vertebral body. This is done with careful X-ray control. Once the needle is in the correct position, bone cement or other substances are squirted down the needle into the vertebral body, stabilizing the fracture. Immediate and lasting pain improvement is customary.

Kyphoplasty

Kyphoplasty is very similar to vertebroplasty except that a larger needle is used, a balloon is passed down the needle, and the balloon is inflated, restoring much of the lost height of the vertebral body. Full height restoration is not possible. The balloon is then deflated and removed, and the resulting empty space is filled with bone cement or a similar substance.

Thoracoplasty

This procedure is usually done in conjunction with a posterior fusion and instrumentation for scoliosis. Instead of taking a bone graft from the pelvis, the surgeon removes pieces of several ribs on the side of the rib prominence ("rib hump"). This technique provides a good source of bone graft and simultaneously reduces the prominence. It takes about six weeks for the ribs to heal solidly.

Pars Interarticularis Repair

The surgeon repairs the basic defect in isthmic spondylolysis. Because only one vertebra is operated on, this procedure is not considered a fusion. This bony defect is located in the pars interarticularis, a piece of bone that connects the lamina of a vertebra to the rest of the vertebra (see Chapter 2). The defect area is exposed through a midline incision (almost always there are defects on both the right and left sides). The soft fibrous tissue in the defect is then removed down to healthy bone, a bone graft (autograft) is applied, and internal fixation is added to hold the bone pieces in place for bone healing. There are several different types of metallic fixation, the choice depending on local anatomy and the surgeon's experience.

Artificial Ligaments

There has been a recent surge in the concept of artificial ligaments to increase the stability of the spine without fusion. These bands of plastic or other synthetic fibers are attached to pedicle screws. The concept is not new, having been tried in the 1980s in both France and the United States. There was no scientific evidence then that artificial ligaments were of any value. Whether the newer type of implants will be more successful remains to be seen.

Interspinous Spacers

These are small pieces of plastic or metal placed in between the spinous processes in the lumbar spine. There is as yet no definite scientific evidence for the value of interspinous spacers. They can be inserted under local anesthesia.

Operations for Chronic Pain

Morphine Pump

The surgeon does a laminectomy, exposes the dura, and places a thin catheter (plastic tube) through the dura against the nerves or spinal cord. This catheter is connected to an implanted pump that delivers a very small but constant dose of morphine. The pump can be refilled by a needle and syringe through the skin. This is very helpful for a majority of patients for which it is used.

Spinal Cord Stimulation

This procedure is for patients with chronic severe pain when nothing else has given them adequate relief. Surgeons have found that the application of tiny electrical impulses directly onto the spinal cord can "block" the pain signals going up the spinal cord to the brain. A surgeon performs a laminectomy, exposes the dura, and places small electrodes on the dural surface. These electrodes are connected to a stimulator device, much like a cardiac pace-maker, buried under the skin. This is usually quite effective.

5

The Twenty-Five Most Common Questions about Back Pain and Its Treatment

1. Is there any way I can prevent back pain?

Anyone can develop back pain, from the very active to the very sedentary. We don't know exactly what causes back pain in every situation. We do know that some activities pose a higher risk for causing back pain. These include heavy lifting and twisting and bending of the trunk. Staying healthy and fit is very important.

2. What medication is best for back pain?

Nonsteroidal antiinflammatory drugs (NSAIDs) are used most often to treat back pain because they have been shown in many scientific studies to give the best relief with the fewest risks. These are discussed in more detail in Chapter 3.

3. Should I use heat or ice when I have back pain?

For the first day or two after the onset of acute back pain, cold therapy (ice or cold packs) usually feels better. After that, heat usually feels better. The warmth helps relax the muscles and ease the spasms.

4. My leg hurts, and my doctor is telling me that the problem is in my back. How can that be?

The nerves to the legs have their origin (the nerve root) in the lumbar spine. When the nerve is pinched or compressed in the spine, it is felt in the leg. You might feel pain, weakness, or numbness.

5. My back pain feels better when I bend forward and is severe when I stand up straight. Why?

Back pain with standing that is alleviated by leaning forward is usually caused by a condition called lumbar spinal stenosis. We often refer to this as the "shopping cart sign." If you have lumbar spinal stenosis, you will feel better when you walk holding onto a shopping cart because as you lean forward, the pressure on the nerves caused by the stenosis is reduced.

6. Why does my back feel better lying down?

You may notice your back pain improves when you lie down. In this position there is less "load" on the discs. Studies have measured the pressure on the discs in different positions. By far, lying down is the position with the least pressure across the disc space.

7. Why do doctors ask me about my bowel and bladder?

The bowel and bladder are controlled by nerves from the spine. If you are having difficulty controlling your bowel and bladder, it might indicate that there is a significant problem in your spinal column. If so, you might need immediate attention and, most likely, emergency surgery.

8. I smoke and my doctor said this can be bad for my back. Why?

Smoking has numerous bad health effects. With respect to the spine, smoking is associated with an increase in osteoporosis. Also, if you are considering surgery that includes a fusion, smoking will interfere with your body's ability to heal after surgery. In fact, there is a 40 % increase in failure of fusion surgery in smokers compared to nonsmokers.

9. I have a torn disc. Will it grow back together?

Once a disc is abnormal, it will always be abnormal. That does not necessarily mean that it will continue to be painful. Most often, a torn and painful disc improves with time and with nonsurgical treatment.

10. I have been diagnosed with degenerative disc disease. Is this hereditary?

There is some evidence that disc degeneration may have a familial tendency. However, a subset of patients have Scheuermann's disease, which can be inherited.

11. I am going to have a disc surgically removed. What will happen to the area where the disc was—the space between the vertebrae?

With routine discectomy, only a small part of the disc is usually re-moved. The remaining part of the disc plus the scar tissue that occurs where part of the disc was removed is enough to provide cushioning between the vertebrae and to keep the vertebrae properly spaced.

12. What is the difference between a discectomy, a laminotomy, and a laminectomy?

A discectomy involves removing part of the disc. A laminotomy mean that part of the lamina (a bony piece of the vertebrae) is sur-gically removed either to relieve pressure on a nerve or to give the surgeon access to a disc herniation. A laminectomy means the entire lamina is removed. A complete laminectomy is seldom necessary for disc herniations, but it is the usual treatment for spinal stenosis.

13. Will taking calcium help my back heal from the fusion I am scheduled to have?

If you eat a balanced diet including the recommended daily intake of calcium, taking more calcium will not help you heal better. However, getting your recommended daily intake of calcium is important for preventing osteoporosis.

14. I have degenerative disc disease. The word *degeneration* makes me think it is going to continue to get worse. What should I expect? Will I ever get better?

Usually when a disc degenerates, it will continue to do so with time. However, a degenerated disc is not always painful. Several studies have shown that many individuals with abnormal discs (as seen on MRI scan) never have back or leg pain. If you have acute onset of lower back pain and are diagnosed with lumbar disc degeneration, there is a good chance most of your symptoms will improve within a year.

15. My doctor recommended a steroid injection. The three I had last month really helped at first, but now my pain is back. Should I go ahead with another injection?

Doctors generally recommend between three and six lumbar epidural steroid injections per year. (In the past, only three were recommended per year.) Too much steroid placed in the same area can cause some local damage, and actually most people do not notice improvement after the third lumbar epidural steroid injection.

16. My doctor recommends a fusion. I hear this procedure can put stress on other parts of my back. Is this true?

When two vertebrae are fused, motion can no longer occur between them. That can place further demands or stress on adjacent discs. It has been thought that this increased stress on adjacent discs can lead to degeneration, but that is not necessarily true. Studies are being done to determine if there is an increase in degeneration above or below a fusion. The final results are not yet available. We do know a single-level fusion does not cause degeneration. There may be an increase in degeneration when multiple levels are fused. Doctors are unsure whether the degeneration is a result of the fusion or if it is due to the natural tendency of the discs to degenerate—that is, the disc would have degenerated with or without the fusion.

17. I have a herniated disc and I am not having surgery. Can I always expect to have back problems?

The diagnosis of a herniated disc does not necessarily mean you will always have back problems. Most people with a herniated disc will notice significant improvement in the first six weeks after symptoms start. In fact, some studies have shown the herniation will actually disappear over time in a small percent of people.

18. What is a rhizotomy?

A rhizotomy is a procedure that destroys a nerve. Most often, radiofrequency is used to do this, but cryotherapy (cold) can be used as well as Botox. This procedure is described in more detail in Chapter 3.

19. What is a TENS unit used for?

A TENS unit uses a gentle electric current to manage chronic back pain. In the spinal cord or brain, the electric current overlaps the painful stimulus, which may provide some pain relief. TENS stands for transcutaneous electrical nerve stimulation and is discussed in Chapter 3.

20. I have osteoporosis. If I have a fusion, will it heal?

Even with osteoporosis, your body can still heal fusions and fractures. The main concern is whether you will be able to hold the internal fixation devices that are used during fusions. With osteo-

6

Adopting the Right M

"Your mindset is everything." It's a favor
coaches and motivational speakers. It's also
those who have discovered that good things a
of their own mental framework.

As someone with back pain, it's important
the power of the right mindset. Your mindset
ble ally in getting the kind of care and treat
help speed your recovery. It can help ke
grounded when your head is swirling with co
and information. And it can chase away helpl
ficult situations.

In short, the right mindset can be one o
tools for better health and quicker healing.

▌ Just What Is a Mindset?

Your mindset is nothing more than the men
proach you bring to any situation or problem

porosis, there is an increase in loosening of the screws that are used to stabilize the spine.

21. Does the instrumentation need to come out of my back once the fusion is healed?

Devices such as screws and rods are often used in spine surgery to help stabilize the spine. The devices are removed in only a small percent of patients. Instrumentation is removed if the screws loosen and cause local irritation and pain or if the prominence of the instrumentation causes a local irritation.

22. I have lumbar spinal stenosis. My doctor ordered an epidural steroid injection. Does that just cover the symptoms? Why not fix it?

Patients with lumbar spinal stenosis are often offered treatment options such as epidural steroid injections before surgery is considered. This is because there is an inflammatory component to the problem in addition to the direct pressure on the nerves. Lumbar epidural steroid injections are usually but not always a temporary measure, and symptoms will frequently return. Your particular situation will dictate the best treatment choice for you. For example, if you have problems that make surgery risky, proceeding with nonsurgical measures to deal with the pain makes sense.

23. I have a disc problem. Why does it hurt so much to sit?

People with disc problems often complain of lower back pain with sitting because the pressure in the disc increases significantly with sitting. Lying down puts the least amount of pressure on the disc, so you might find relief from your pain in that position.

24. I was given narcotic medications for my back pain. I am afraid to take them. What if I get addicted?

Narcotic medication is frequently used f
tial treatment of severe lower back and leg p
for addiction, even with a short prescrip
should be used very carefully. As a patient,
the risk involved in taking them.

25. Is surgery effective for treating lowe

Until several years ago, surgery for lowe
fective than it is today because surgical an
were not optimal. Recent advances in perfor
cally treating discs have dramatically increas
cal treatment for lower back pain. With prop
optimal surgical techniques, the success rat
gery for back pain is now about 90%. Doct
back pain cannot be treated surgically simpl
the latest advances and outcomes in surgery

*Special thanks to Dr. Manuel Pinto for hi
chapter.*

ple don't realize that there are two different sides to this coin: (1) what we think and feel and (2) what we present to others.

Your mindset has less to do with the specifics of a given situation than it does with how you react and respond to it. Let's use the weather as an example. Joe hates snow. As soon as the white fluffy stuff starts falling, Joe slips into a foul mood. He associates snow with heavy shoveling, snarled traffic, and bulky winter coats. In contrast, Leticia loves snow. She associates snow with crisp, refreshing walks followed by relaxing evenings in front of the fire. When Leticia sees snow, she perks up. Both people are experiencing the same situation—falling snow—but their mindsets are radically different.

When we talk about adopting the right mindset, we mean taking an approach that increases your chances of getting what you need and arriving at the best possible outcome. Your mindset thus relates to every health care professional with whom you meet or speak, any type of treatment you undertake, every medical decision you make, and, of course, to yourself, your back, your pain, and your healing and recovery.

Right now you probably have lots of thoughts and feelings—many of them not very pleasant—about your back pain and the ways that it has affected your life. Maybe you're frustrated at having to live with the pain as long as you have. Or maybe you're angry about getting hurt in the first place. If you've already tried multiple treatments and haven't gotten better, you might be feeling fear or despair. It is okay to feel any or even all of these things. Having the right mindset is not about somehow cheering up, ignoring your pain, or pretending that things are different from how they actually are. We're not talking about doing some rah-rah self-talk or telling yourself to just buck up.

The right mindset is much bigger and far more effective than this. It is a practical tool that can be used to help you and to improve your situation. In this chapter, you'll learn how to use this tool to your best advantage.

A helpful mindset has three important elements: *empowerment, optimism,* and *fortitude*. In combination, these elements create a powerful force for helping others do their best for you and for helping you do the most for yourself. Let's look at each of these elements briefly.

Empowerment

Empowerment is the belief that you have the ability and resources to bring about the best possible outcome—becoming free of back pain. And you truly *do* have all of this because you have this book guiding you.

Empowerment does not allow you to give up, settle for second best, or be pushed in a direction you don't want to go. It does not let you play the role of the passive sick person. Instead, empowerment pushes you to find the situations and solutions that feel right and work best for you.

Other people respond to how you present yourself; they cannot read your mind. Presenting a mindset of empowerment to others markedly influences how they interact with you. An empowered mindset can regularly tilt interactions with others in your favor.

Optimism

Optimism is the potent combination of positiveness and hope. Again, you have every reason to feel both of these because you have this book coaching you every step of the way and because you've embraced empowerment instead of passivity.

Optimism is choosing to believe that good things can and will happen—not in every single moment, of course, but often. Optimism says, "Things may be very difficult right now, but I believe they can and will get better." When you present an optimistic mindset to others, you encourage them to do their best for you, to like you, and to also feel more optimistic about your situation.

Most important of all, optimistic people are more likely to recover from illness and pain, they tend to heal faster, and they are less likely to have a reoccurrence of the same health problem later on. We now have plenty of studies that show optimism does make a profound difference in people's health. (If you want to know more about some of these studies, read Martin Seligman's book *Learned Optimism*.)

Fortitude

Fortitude is simply the ability and the willingness to cope with whatever circumstances come your way. It doesn't mean liking them, or never complaining about them, or never getting upset about them. But it does mean accepting them, handling them, and being willing to do what needs to be done.

Your path to healing and freedom from back pain may have ups and downs, and your recovery may proceed in fits and starts. Fortitude enables you to hang in when the going gets tough or frustrating. It allows you to be patient with the process, with those around you, and with yourself.

▌Putting the Right Mindset to Work

Almost everyone has had at least one negative experience with a medical professional. While the right mindset is not a money-back guarantee that all your interactions with doctors and other health care workers will go smoothly, it can dramatically increase the possibility of getting you what you want and need.

So, for starters, bring empowerment with you every time you see or speak with a medical professional. Expect to be taken seriously, to be respected, and to be treated like the valued client you are.

(This is no less true if you are visiting a free public clinic or hospital.) If you have any question or need more information at any time, ask for it. If you don't fully understand an explanation, ask for more detail. If you still don't understand, ask to be directed to a good source of information such as a consumer reference book or a website for nonprofessionals.

Notice that empowerment does not mean being suspicious, guarded, or defensive, and it certainly does not mean expecting incompetence in others. Instead, it's a combination of curiosity, calm, confidence, and active participation.

Whenever you see or speak with any medical professional, bring optimism with you, too. Expect a positive experience. This is entirely realistic if you've had a good experience with this person before or if you're seeing him or her for the first time. (Remember, most medical professionals are good at what they do, or they wouldn't be able to keep their jobs.) And if you've had a negative experience with someone before, don't see that person again! Instead, insist on working with someone different.

When you're optimistic, most people will pick up on your optimism and respond more positively toward you. So stay open, friendly, and cooperative unless you feel that someone is not listening to you or acting in your best interests.

For the most part, the era of the small, friendly neighborhood clinic or hospital is gone. Most clinics and hospitals are now part of huge health care systems. Interacting with these systems, even when their employees have the best training and intentions, can leave you feeling a bit like a product on an assembly line. This is where fortitude can be so helpful. Each system, and each clinic and hospital, will have its own procedures, forms, and etiquette. Everyone who works there will be familiar with all of these, but—at least at first—all of it will be new to you. Be patient with yourself as you learn how the system works and how to get it to work for you. Ask for help—repeatedly if necessary. If anything is confusing or unclear, ask again. If necessary, say, "I'm new here, and I'm used to doing things differently, so I'm getting confused. Can you tell me exactly what I need to do next and what will happen after I do it?"

Some final words on fortitude: When you tell others that your back hurts, they will think you're wearing a big sign that says, "Please give me advice!" Almost everybody will have an opinion—possibly a very strong one—about the best treatment or course of action. Typically, these opinions will contradict one another. (For instance, one person may tell you that a chiropractor is the only answer, whereas another may dismiss all chiropractors as quacks.) As you are deluged with all this free advice, fortitude is the order of the day. The truth is that most people will not have any real idea what you are going through—and few will realize that a hurting back can have many different causes, each one requiring a different form of treatment. Nevertheless, remind yourself that their advice is an expression of their caring about you. Be patient with them. Listen to what they say and thank them for their suggestions. Then keep following the guidance in this book.

Treat yourself with patience, fortitude, and respect as well. It's easy to get down on yourself if you're not healing as quickly as you'd like or if you make a mistake and reaggravate your back. Cut yourself some slack. Mistakes happen, and life is full of unknowns. Throughout your healing and recovery, treat yourself with the same care and respect that you expect from others. It's not just what you deserve—it's also one of the best things you can do for your back.

▌ The Right Mindset Equals Reduced Pain

Here's one other way in which your mindset is important: it can directly reduce or increase your back pain. Muscles are often major contributors to back pain. When you are stressed out or tense, your muscles may tighten, causing increased pain. If you worry unnecessarily, obsess over little things, or cling to your worries and fears, the resulting stress can cause increased muscle tension. In contrast, empowerment, optimism, and fortitude can lessen stress, leading to relaxed muscles and diminished pain.

▌ Ten Tips for Developing the Most Beneficial Mindset ▌

1. **Participate actively in every aspect of your treatment and healing.** Never consider yourself a passive sick person to be healed by experts. And never let yourself be bullied or shamed into silence or compliance.

2. **Consider yourself the most essential part of your health care team,** one that includes all the professionals who are helping you recover. (Why are you the most essential member? Because no one has better information about how your back feels than you do.)

3. **Once you've found people you trust, show them that trust, work with them, and let them do their jobs.** They are your partners in healing, not adversaries to be watched with suspicion. (And if you don't trust someone, don't work with that person. Trust is essential in any health care relationship, so if trust isn't there, by all means find someone else.)

4. **Stay focused and attentive in any discussion you have with a health care professional.** Careful, attentive listening will help you better understand your situation, your options, and the risks and benefits of each. It will help you be informed rather than confused, and it will help you cut through any myths or potential misunderstandings. Your own health is at stake, so this is no time to multitask or daydream. After a complex or detailed discussion, we also recommend requesting a written summary that you can review later on.

5. **Become informed and ask questions.** Learn more about the sp⁻ and the back. Once you have a diagnosis, learn mo⁻

your condition. Ask for the names of good books and websites. Most medical professionals will have free pamphlets that describe your condition, possible treatments, how your recovery will proceed, and so on. And always—*always*—ask questions about anything you don't understand.

6. **Pay attention to your body.** Notice what hurts and what feels good. Then make sure you pass on that information to medical professionals with as much clarity and detail as you can.

7. **Don't let anyone else make your medical decisions for you.** There may be more than one good way to treat your condition. If so, only *you* can (and should) choose the right treatment. Don't ask medical professionals to decide for you (though you certainly can ask for their recommendations and advice). And don't let family members or anyone else pressure you into a making a decision that's not in your own best interests.

8. **Pick your medical professionals carefully.** Ask for referrals to the best and most experienced people. Learn about each professional's experience and training.

9. **Schedule a second session to sit down and talk before deciding on any surgery.** When surgery is first mentioned as an option, you may have a strong emotional reaction. As a result, you may take in little of what the physician tells you. A second discussion—one that takes place after you've had a chance to process earlier information and consider a variety of options—can be extremely helpful and empowering. We suggest doing the following:

- Come to this meeting with a written list of questions.
- Listen to all answers attentively, taking notes if necessary.
- Ask for details or for a referral to helpful resources if there's anything you don't understand.
- Request a written summary of information about the surgery from the physician.

10. **Remember that medicine is an art as much as a science.** Sometimes the right diagnosis or best treatment is not easy or obvious. Sometimes medical professionals will disagree. Sometimes the best they can do is make intelligent guesses. But this is true of almost everything in life. Remind yourself that medical professionals are human beings just like you.

The right mindset undergirds everything we talk about in the remaining chapters. In fact, most of these chapters focus on applying the right mindset in a wide range of situations with a variety of people.

In a sense, everything we've said here about mindset boils down to two simple words: *take charge*. By taking charge of your mindset, your condition, and your own healing and recovery, you maximize your chances for reclaiming a healthy back as quickly as possible.

7

The Benefits of Taking Charge and the Costs of Being Passive

In the previous chapter, you learned why the right mindset toward your own healing, treatment, and recovery is so essential. Yet a good mindset alone isn't enough. It must be translated into practical, self-aware action.

When you're dealing simultaneously with pain, uncertainty, multiple options, and sometimes-confusing medical advice, it's extremely tempting to tell yourself the doctor knows what's best and to do whatever the doctor recommends. We've written this chapter to show you why resisting this temptation is so important.

The two stories that follow are accurate accounts of what happened to Dr. Bach. Each involved a serious health problem, and each required her to make a number of important health care decisions.

In the first story, she unquestioningly followed the advice, referrals, and treatments that she was offered in good faith by medical professionals. The results nearly killed her.

In the second—which involves the treatment and cure of severe back pain—she took charge of her own healing from the very beginning. Throughout her treatment and recovery, she asked questions, researched her options, and oversaw the creation of a customized recovery plan ideally suited for her. The result was a quick and complete return to health and vitality.

Read the two stories that follow and take them to heart. If at any time in your own healing journey you find yourself feeling embarrassed, squeamish, or worried about challenging medical authority (or members of your own family), read both stories again. Then speak up.

▌ Baa, Baa, Bach Sheep: The Costs of Passivity

I learned the hard way how important it is to choose the right health care professionals. In fact, I learned that making the right choice could save your life; making the wrong one almost killed me several years ago.

It's funny. If I'd wanted to buy a new car or even a new washing machine, I would have thoroughly checked out the different makes and models with *Consumer Reports* magazine and done a good deal of research on the web. Yet when it came to my own health and well-being, I didn't do the slightest bit of research or comparison shopping. As a result, I had major surgery without checking out my surgeon's credentials.

It began like this: On a fine August evening, a friend treated me to a sumptuous dinner: stuffed lobster dipped in melted butter capped off with a homemade ice cream cake topped with whipped cream.

A few hours later, at 2:00 A.M., I was awakened by excruciating pain in my chest. I fell on the floor, grasping at my chest and crying out in pain. I thought I was having a heart attack.

After a bit, I was able to sit up. I phoned my family physician and described my pain in detail. He asked me about my recent activities, and I told him about my extravagant, fat-laden dinner. He told me I was probably having a gallbladder attack. He asked me to come in for an exam the next morning and said that I didn't need to run to the emergency room.

He examined me in his office eight hours later. My EKG (electro-cardiogram) was normal, so he referred me to a local surgeon he knew for a more detailed evaluation. I called the surgeon and made an appointment. *(Mistake #1: I failed to ask my physician anything about the surgeon.)*

I met with the surgeon, who examined me further and recom-mended immediate laparoscopic surgery for the removal of my gall-bladder. *(Mistakes #2 through #7: I didn't ask the surgeon any of these questions:*

- *Why do I have to have surgery immediately?*
- *How many laparoscopic gallbladder removals have you per-formed?*
- *What is the rate of complications for this surgery?*
- *What are the potential dangers?*
- *Are any other treatment options available?*
- *How potentially effective—and dangerous—is each one?)*

In laparoscopic surgery, a thin tube is inserted into the patient's abdomen through a small incision in the skin, and tissue or organs are removed through it. This differs from the more traditional "open" surgery, in which a much larger incision is made. Laparo-scopic surgery also differs in another important way: it has its own unique set of possible—and possibly deadly—complications.

The surgeon recommended laparoscopic surgery because of the usually short recovery time and the reduced amount of scarring. But he told me nothing about potential dangers and complications. He also did not mention that, like many surgeons in 1997, he had rela-tively little experience with that form of surgery.

Instead of spending an hour or two researching laparoscopic

surgery—and the surgeon himself—in my hurry to avoid further pain I made *mistake #8: I said yes right then and there in his office.*

Early the next week, I was admitted to a local hospital and the surgeon performed supposedly routine laparoscopic gallbladder surgery on me. The operation was deemed a success, and I was sent home to recover.

But I didn't recover. Over the next two weeks, I failed to regain either strength or energy. I saw the surgeon again for a postsurgical exam. I told him about my lack of energy and strength, but after giving me a brief standard physical, he declared my condition to be normal postsurgical fatigue. *(Mistake #9: I failed to challenge him on this or ask him about it, even though I am normally a very outgoing person.)*

Several more weeks passed. I still felt very weak and tired, but I continued to tell myself *(mistake #10)* that I was recovering slowly but normally.

Three months after the operation, I saw my diligent family physician (not the surgeon) for a routine postsurgical follow-up exam that he had requested. The exam included a battery of blood tests.

The results of the tests immediately alarmed my physician, who ordered an ultrasound of my liver. The blood tests showed that my alkaline phosphatase was *over 100 times* normal and indicated severe liver damage or malfunction. The ultrasound that followed revealed more than a *quart* of bile in my peritoneum (a membrane in the abdomen that covers the internal organs and creates a potential cavity in which fluids can collect).

To better diagnose the problem, that same afternoon I had the first of many CAT (computerized axial tomography) scans. The scan showed that the bile duct system leading from my liver had inadvertently been damaged during the gallbladder surgery.

Since I had liver damage, obviously the right thing to do at this point was to see a liver and bile duct surgical specialist. Yet I didn't *(mistake #11)*. Instead, with my liver (and my life) at risk, I chose to go back to the surgeon who had botched the original operation and to my family physician. I was presented with these options:

1. Drain the bile from the peritoneum. This step was essential regardless of whatever else would be done.
2. Seal the part of the bile duct system now leaking into my peritoneum through a minimally invasive procedure. I was told by the surgeon that this surgery posed little risk and had a reasonable chance of working. *(Mistake #12: I did not ask about the risks, complications, and success rates for this option.)*
3. Do nothing and hope that the leak would seal itself. This was possible but unlikely—and it certainly hadn't happened so far.
4. Seal off the damaged part of the bile duct system through major surgery. The surgeon told me that this was the option most likely to succeed, but it also involved the highest risk and was the most potentially debilitating surgery.

At this point, I finally realized that I needed to stop letting others make my medical decisions for me. I began gathering more information. I consulted with my son, who is a physician, and he answered many of my questions. After some thought, I chose drainage of the bile, plus the less-invasive form of surgery.

I was fitted with a peritoneal drain, which drained bile out through a hole in my waist, and several weeks later I had the small-scale procedure performed by a team recommended by both my physician and the surgeon who had caused the original problem *(mistake #13)*.

The surgery failed. Bile continued to drain into my abdomen.

Doctors now know that the best surgical results are usually achieved by surgeons who specialize in a very specific area—in this case, the liver and bile ducts—and who perform the surgery in a hospital that has lots of experience in that medical subspecialty. Unfortunately, no one told me this, though I might have discovered it for myself if I had done some basic research *(mistake #14)*.

At this point, I decided that input from specialists was in order. This meant spending money on doctor visits not fully covered by my health insurance. But by now the issue was saving my life, not saving money.

I decided to go to the Mayo Clinic in Rochester, Minnesota, for further assessment and treatment. All the experts at Mayo agreed that part of my bile duct system had been severed. The Mayo team recommended that I continue wearing the peritoneal drain but that it should be repositioned to function more effectively. Their hope was that the damaged part of my bile duct system would then close on its own, stopping the flow of bile to my peritoneum.

The Mayo doctors repositioned the drain several times, but with each passing week I became weaker and more discouraged. By the eighteenth week after my initial surgery, I was so fatigued that I couldn't cook for myself, bathe myself, or walk 30 feet to my mailbox. Only a limited amount of home health care was provided by my insurance, so I tapped my savings to hire someone to help me in my home.

About a month later, the drainage finally stopped. The bile duct had resealed itself, and there was no more bile in my abdomen. Five months after the peritoneal drain had been inserted and nearly eight months after the initial surgery, I could now begin my recovery. However, I was weak, demoralized, and out twenty thousand dollars for specialists and home health care.

Returning to my formerly active self required months of rehabilitative physical therapy. And it was three years after my initial gallbladder surgery that I finally returned to full health.

I sued the surgeon who had botched the gallbladder operation. But I lost; the court determined that my surgeon's inadvertent nicking of the bile duct system was within the normal range of medical complications for that procedure.

■ A Patient with Backbone: The Benefits of Taking Charge

Fortunately, I am old (and stubborn) enough to learn from my mistakes. So when I unexpectedly needed treatment and ultimately surgery for a back problem a couple of years later, I knew I had to take a completely different approach.

From the beginning, I took an active role, asking questions, researching the relevant topics, and insisting on being the central decision maker at every stage of my treatment and recovery. Most important of all, I chose all of my health care professionals extremely carefully. My successful recovery was guided by careful and thorough research into the appropriate people, treatments, and options.

The problems began in December 2000 when I dragged a heavy suitcase down my winding back stairs and hauled it into my car. For the next six hours, as I drove to a ski resort, sharp pains intermittently pierced my left leg. I worried that I had somehow injured it.

My first step was to be examined thoroughly by my regular physician. After lab tests ruled out infection and cancer, he concluded that a back injury was the source of the searing leg pain. I asked him what he recommended, and he suggested a regimen of physical therapy. I immediately asked *(smart move #1)*, "Who is the most experienced physical therapist in the Twin Cities—the PT with the best track record for treating patients with back pain?"

My doctor referred me to Eve Russell, who quickly put me on physical therapy, as well as a modified Pilates program, to stretch and build my abdominal and back muscles. I spent several months doing physical therapy and Pilates. I also began doing some focused reading on the subject of back self-care *(smart move #2)*. I found

Robin McKenzie's book *Treat Your Own Back* especially valuable. McKenzie's program is primarily a series of extension exercises aimed at "centralizing" back pain—moving the pain from the leg (or legs) to the midback. McKenzie also recommends certain sleeping positions and the use of a lumbar roll (a rolling pin–like object placed behind the back) for prolonged sitting, such as while driving. I did McKenzie's exercises, used the lumbar roll in my car, and adopted one of his sleeping positions; all of these did help my back somewhat.

Still, after several months of PT, Pilates, McKenzie's exercises, and nonsteroidal pain medication (ibuprofen and Aleve), my back still bothered me. I told my physician, who suggested that an evaluation by an orthopedic surgeon was in order.

But before even agreeing to be evaluated by an orthopedic surgeon, I sought recommendations. I asked my doctor, Eve Russell, and several other physical therapists to recommend the orthopedic surgeon who, in their mind, had both lots of experience and the most successful track record for cases similar to mine *(smart move #3)*. In each case, I also asked whether the surgeon they recommended was certified by the American Board of Orthopedic Surgery *(smart move #4)*. Interestingly, everyone recommended the Twin Cities Spine Center, and three people recommended Dr. Joseph Perra (who wrote the introduction to this book) in particular. Soon afterward, I made an appointment with Dr. Perra.

Before my appointment, however, I put together the following list of questions for Dr. Perra *(smart move #5)*:

- Is your primary focus treating back problems? (Desired answer: yes.)
- Are you comfortable with an approach that doesn't involve surgery? (Desired answer: yes.)
- Will you exhaust all nonsurgical avenues before recommending surgery? (Desired answer: yes.)

- Can you tell me how often and for how long I will need to be treated? (I desired a clear, specific treatment plan that both sounded and felt sensible.)

At my appointment, I not only asked these questions but watched for the following warning signs, either of which, had Dr. Perra done them, would have given me serious doubts about his trustworthiness *(smart move #6)*:

- Suggested a treatment before completing a full physical exam, taking a complete history, and reviewing all my tests and studies
- Discouraged me from getting a second opinion

Dr. Perra passed all of my tests with flying colors. He did a thorough physical exam, evaluated my gait, looked at my X-rays, answered all my questions completely, and raised none of the warning flags listed above.

His diagnosis was not one problem but three: (1) degenerative disc disease, (2) spondylosis (degenerative changes due to osteoarthritis), and (3) radiculopathy (a compression of the nerve roots in the spine).

Dr. Perra felt that surgery wasn't appropriate yet. Instead, he suggested a back physical therapy program (including an exercise ball) and nonsteroidal pain medication. He urged me to try this for six weeks, then to meet with him again.

The PT program involved stretching and strengthening my abdominal and back muscles. However, I was to use a large ball rather than floor exercises. I was also to supplement this with walking and with riding an exercise bike.

To my surprise, the program worked. It kept my back pain-free for the next two years. Surgery was neither necessary nor even discussed.

Then, in the fall of 2002, the leg pain suddenly returned, triggered by the same causes (hauling a heavy suitcase, followed by hours of driving). This time, however, the pain was in both legs.

I sought help once again. I went back to both my regular physician and Eve Russell, the PT. I was put on several months of physical therapy, but it did not bring me either pain relief or improved leg function.

My doctor prescribed the analgesic Darvocet and a stronger analgesic combination, Tylenol with codeine. Later, my physician also prescribed Celebrex, a prescription-strength antiinflammatory medication. Although all helped somewhat, they did not provide adequate relief.

Meanwhile, my left foot had become numb as well and could no longer be depended on. Twice, while walking my dog, the leg suddenly buckled and I fell.

I knew it was time to start climbing the pyramid again.

With my physician's blessing, I went to see Dr. Perra once again *(smart move #7)*. Both doctors agreed that it was time to try another approach. Dr. Perra suggested a short trial of cortisone injections into my spine to reduce inflammation. These injections would need to be given by a radiologist.

I asked for a referral from Dr. Perra's office—but not just any referral; I insisted on seeing the radiologist whom Dr. Perra personally ranked the highest *(smart move #8)*.

I was happy with the radiologist, and the first cortisone injection helped for a few weeks. But the second injection, administered a month later, created extreme, searing pain in my left leg. Only a strong dose of Oxycontin (a powerful narcotic) enabled me to get through the night.

The next morning, I was unable to put any weight on my left leg, and my blood pressure was dangerously high. I went to the emergency room at University Hospital in Minneapolis, where the medical team was able to lower my pain and blood pressure with intravenous morphine. The attending physician team strongly recommended a surgical consultation as soon as possible.

Shortly thereafter, I made new appointments with Dr. Perra and my regular physician *(smart move #9)*. All three of us agreed that it was time to have surgery.

But I insisted that other forms of care accompany the surgery *(smart move #10)*. I discussed preoperative preparations with Eve Russell. I asked her to help me prepare my body for the limitations of recovery from surgery such as difficulty getting in and out of bed. She taught me to do log rolls from and into bed, as well as several other exercises to help me build my upper body strength. All of these proved immensely helpful in the weeks that followed.

I saw Dr. Perra once again as well. He examined me thoroughly, ordered an MRI (magnetic resonance imaging), and then suggested decompression surgery, which he would perform himself. Yet before I agreed to surgery, I asked for a good deal of specific information and insisted on responses in writing *(smart move #11):*

- How will the operation work? What will you do in it? (Answer: My pain was caused by pressure on a nerve. Dr. Perra would remove a portion of the bone overlaying the compressed nerve and trace the nerve out to make certain it was free from pressure. This operation is known as a decompressive laminectomy.)
- What are the risks? (Answer: a small chance of damage to one or more nerves; the usual low-level risks associated with anesthesia, bleeding, muscle trauma, and infection; a small risk that the surgery would offer only short-term relief or no relief at all.)
- What scars or other physical evidence of the operation will remain afterward? (Answer: I would have a scar about 5 inches long on my spine.)
- How long will recovery likely take? (Answer: several weeks to three months.)

- What will I need to do during recovery? (Answer: wear a back brace for several weeks and do some rehabilitation therapy after my initial recuperation at home.)

Dr. Perra provided complete, clear answers. Still, I made a point of asking him for a referral to another PT *(smart move #12)*. Eve Russell was very good, but I wanted a physical therapist who had extensive experience with people healing from decompression surgery. I also wanted the one person whom Dr. Perra and his staff trusted the most for postoperative PT. He gave me the name of Cate Pandiscio. Only after I had spoken to her and was convinced that she was as good as Dr. Perra said did I schedule the surgery *(smart move #13)*.

My surgery was a complete and rousing success. On the first day afterward, I was able to walk with a walker. By day two, to everyone's surprise, I was walking up and down the hospital corridor with ease. By day three, I was walking briskly through the hospital corridors and negotiating the hospital stairs. Two days later, I was home.

Following a postoperative checkup with Dr. Perra, I began a course of physical therapy with Cate Pandiscio. I soon learned that Cate herself had had successful back surgery performed by a member of the Twin Cities Spine Center. I saw Cate for eight weeks, easily performing the strengthening, stretching, and balancing exercises she assigned me, as well as the three short walks (instead of one longer walk) per day that we both felt would be helpful.

After eight weeks of PT with Cate, she told me that I no longer showed any signs of having had back surgery. I had regained my strength and balance in a remarkably short time. Cate told me that going into surgery healthy, fit, and knowledgeable had made a tremendous positive difference for me.

It has been two years since my surgery. I am pain-free and strong, and I have good balance. I walk briskly 20 to 25 miles per week and perform a challenging strengthening and stretching exercise routine three to four times per week. My back feels great. Best of all, I feel confident about being able to stay focused and in charge of my own healing, no matter what may come my way.

▌ It's Your Call

This book isn't just about good ideas and smart mindsets. It's about your own back, your own pain, and your own healing.

In this chapter, you've read about two serious health conditions, two very different ways of approaching them, and two completely different sets of outcomes.

At any point—regardless of what others tell you and what you may have done (or not done) before—you have a choice: the path of passivity or the path of advocacy, assertiveness, and self-care.

The events described in this chapter strikingly bring home the need to approach your health care in a systematic way. This experience led us to the development of the Back Care Pyramid. The Back Care Pyramid is a rational, easy-to-understand guide to the various levels of care that can be used to treat back pain.

The base of the pyramid is self-care, the easiest and least expensive pathway. Most people with back pain can solve their problems at this level.

If that does not work, the next step is to see your family doctor. He or she will ask you some questions, do a physical examination, perhaps do some tests, and then make a recommendation. Depending on the findings, this might be a medication, a referral to a physical therapist, a request for more specialized testing, or a referral to a specialist.

If the family physician is unable to solve your problem, then a referral up the pyramid is appropriate. The next level is the specialist.

The Back Care Pyramid

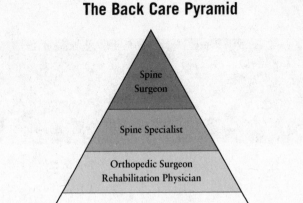

Spine
Surgeon

Spine Specialist

Orthopedic Surgeon
Rehabilitation Physician

Family/Primary Care Doctor

Self-Care

This might be one of several types of specialists who deal with back pain problems, including orthopedic surgeons, neurosurgeons, neurologists, and physiatrists (specialists in physical medicine and rehabilitation). These specialists devote 80% to 90% of their practice to their area of specialty.

The next level up the pyramid is the spine specialist, a physician who devotes at least 80% to 90% of his or her practice to back problems. At the highest level of the pyramid is the spine surgeon, who may be either an orthopedic spine surgeon or a neurosurgical spine surgeon. The key is that he or she devotes 80% to 90% of his or her practice to the spine. It is very important to remember that just because you are referred to a spine surgeon, it does not necessarily mean that you will have surgery.

Do you always have to go up the pyramid one step at a time? No. There are certain situations where surgery is the only answer, and for these very special circumstances you go straight to the top. Chapter 12 discusses the pyramid in much greater detail.

8

Self-Care

The most important pathway of treatment is what you do for yourself. It is the first step of the Back Care Pyramid. There are two parts to this management system: the physical and the mental. The physical things relate to what activities you should do and not do, heat and cold, any medicines you might take, sleeping and resting positions, and exercises. The mental things relate to your ability to avoid depression, to maintain a positive mindset, and to understand the normal evolution of your problem.

▌ Acute Back Pain

Although most acute back pain is located in the lower back area (lumbar spine), problems can occur in the neck and upper back. As we have said earlier, the neck is a special problem and is not discussed in this book. Acute back pain can occur as a result of a fall, from lifting something heavy, from twisting or bending, from coughing or vomiting violently, or from doing nothing at all.

About 90% of acute back pain problems are the result of some kind of stress to the spine. In the past, these were labeled as muscle strains or as back sprains without any specific test to exactly determine the cause. Currently, there is a strong feeling that most of these problems are disc disorders. Regardless of the cause, there is the onset of muscle spasms, which are of themselves painful. This is important to know, since simply the knowledge that you are miserable because of muscle spasms means that most of the time simple measures plus tincture of time will result in your becoming comfortable.

What exactly should you do? Let us take for example a man who yesterday helped his neighbor move a lot of heavy furniture. This morning, he woke up with back pain, was barely able to get out of bed, and couldn't go to work at his regular job. Should he call his doctor? Should he go to the chiropractor? Is there something he can do for himself?

The five key self-treatments are (1) resting in the contour position (see Fig. 1, p. 8); (2) putting cold packs on the back for the first twenty-four hours and then switching to heat; (3) taking over-the counter pain medicines (aspirin, acetaminophen, or ibuprofen) in the recommended doses; (4) avoiding heavy lifting, twisting, and bending; and (5) keeping a positive mindset.

What should you not do? Don't just keep on doing the things that got you into trouble in the first place. Don't move or lift things until you feel better. If your trouble began after twisting your back on the golf course, don't try to play golf until you're much better. Don't call you doctor and ask for narcotics so that you can just keep going. Prescription narcotics are dangerous, both because of their addictive tendencies and because you shouldn't drive a car while taking them.

Don't rush off to the chiropractor until you have given the simple, basic things a good try. Chiropractic has a good track record for acute pain problems but a poor track record for making a specific diagnosis. Why see any doctor if you can cure the problem yourself?

▌ Subacute Back Pain

Now you've done a good job of getting over that acute attack and are feeling much better, but you're not 100% okay. At this point, you should not be spending your time in bed. *Don't be a couch potato!* For acute attacks, only two to three days of bed rest are recommended. You need to get moving. Walking is an excellent way to begin your rehabilitation. You should start slowly with two or three short walks rather than one long walk. As you progress, the length of each walk should increase gradually, and your speed of walking should also increase. It's okay to lie down in the contour position for a little while after each walk.

Minimize the time you spend sitting. It's actually harder on the back than standing, since there are many more muscles being used while standing than sitting. Studies of the pressure inside a disc show it to be higher while sitting as compared to standing. If you're standing to do some work, put one foot up on a box. This further reduces your swayback and gives more comfort.

Another good way to get exercise without hurting your back is to use a swimming pool if one is available. The water takes away the effect of gravity and allows you to use your muscles without stressing the spine.

Now is the time to begin slowly to get into an exercise program that will help your back. Exercises are discussed in Chapter 15. Flexion exercises work best for some people, and extension exercises are better for others. Find out which ones work best for you.

Now is also the time to work on those other things that contribute to your back problem—for example, weight problems and bad habits such as smoking and excessive alcohol intake. These things can't be changed overnight, but you have to start sometime, and it might as well be now.

▮ Chronic Back Pain

If you've had significant (enough to interfere with your daily activities) back pain for more than a couple of months, you are in the chronic phase of back pain. You need to get professional help. You cannot treat this condition on your own. Contact you primary care doctor and get an evaluation. It is important to get a diagnosis, which means getting the answer to why you are hurting.

9

Using the Internet

The Internet is a wonderful tool, allowing its users ready access to an abundance of information. You can research almost any topic on the Internet including back problems and how they are treated. But how good is the information you get on the Internet? When it comes to your back problem and your health, this is a very important question.

If you focus on the best websites, the Internet can be an excellent tool in helping you understand your back problem. The Internet cannot specifically diagnose your particular problem. Your doctor must do that. It is okay to use the Internet to find good information about back problems, but rely on your doctor for help in specifically evaluating, diagnosing, and treating your particular back condition.

▌ Information Overload

Recently, I (Dr. Winter) typed "back pain" into the Google search engine on several occasions. (A search engine is a way to find or access information on the Internet.) Between 12 million and 22 million websites came up; that is, the Internet had over 12 million different places to get information on back pain. When I limited the search to lower back pain, I got between 8 million and 12 million sites. Talk about information overload!

If I spent just five minutes looking at each website for twelve hours each day, it would take me more than two hundred fifty years to look at them all. How can anyone find useful information about their specific back problem in this sea of information?

To get you started in the right direction, we have developed some simple guidelines for finding the most helpful Internet sources for reliable and safe information about back pain. In addition, we have listed some of the best websites for information on health and back pain.

Website Addresses

Every website has a specific address. The address tells the search engine where to go on the Internet to find the site you are looking for. Almost every address starts with the initials *www*, which stand for "world wide web." More important, every address ends with one of three sets of initials: .com, .org, or .edu. The ending initials tell you a lot about the website.

• .com is short for commercial. These sites are sponsored by organizations that seek to make money from the Internet. At first glance, they might look informational or educational, but a closer look reveals more. A good example is www.spine-health.com. This website offers some good general information about what causes back pain, how it can be treated, and recent research about this topic. This site is sponsored by two of the largest sellers of spine implants: Medtronic and Johnson & Johnson. You wouldn't know that by looking at the website address. Another example is www.back.com. This site is sponsored by Medtronic. It offers to help you find a doctor in your area, but it only lists surgeons who use Medtronic products.

- .org is short for organization. An Internet address that ends with these initials is sponsored by a nonprofit organization or a professional organization such as the American Academy of Orthopedic Surgeons. These organizations use the Internet to provide information and are not selling anything.

- .edu is short for education. Internet addresses that end in .edu are sponsored by universities. Again, their goal is to provide information, not to sell you something.

Websites with addresses ending with .org or .edu are the best places to look for information on back problems. The worst places to look are the .com sites.

The Best Websites for Information on Back Problems

Websites sponsored by reputable medical organizations are some of the best sources of Internet information on back problems. The information in this chapter is by no means complete, but it will give you some good places to begin.

The website of the American Academy of Family Practice, www.aafp.org, is one of the very best. It provides general facts about acute back pain, how to tell if your back problem requires emergency help, causes of back pain, and the customary tests and treatments for various back problems.

The website of the American Academy of Orthopedic Surgeons, www.orthoinfo.aaos.org, is another good one. This website lists various conditions and parts of the skeleton, so you need to go to the section on the spine and back pain. This site covers why lower back pain is common, how it is diagnosed, when surgery may be helpful, and what exercises may be useful.

The North American Spine Society website, www.spine.org, is

the site for medical specialists who devote the majority of their practice to spine problems. Medical specialists include those in orthopedic surgery, neurosurgery, neurology, physical medicine and rehabilitation, and radiology.

The website of the Scoliosis Research Society, www.srs.com, has excellent information on many kinds of back problems, not just scoliosis.

The website for the Scoliosis Association, Inc., is scoliosis-assoc.org. This is the lay group for scoliosis and other spine problems and can be very helpful to those with questions and concerns.

Finally, the website of the American Association of Neurological Surgeons, www.neurosurgery.org, is another source of reliable information on back problems.

Most of the good .edu websites for back problem information are sponsored by university medical centers. Some good ones are

- www.healthcare.ucla.edu, the website of the University of California at Los Angeles
- www.orthop.washington.edu, the website of the orthopedic department at the University of Washington, Seattle
- www.lib.uiowa.edu, the website of the University of Iowa

One exception to the .edu rule is the Mayo Clinic. Its website is www.mayoclinic.com only because it is a private enterprise and not a university. The Mayo Clinic has its own medical school and its website has excellent information on virtually every health topic including back problems.

As we noted before, the worst place to search for information on your back problem is the commercial websites—those that end with .com (with the exception of the Mayo Clinic as noted). For example, http://my.webmd.com is the Web MD Health website. It contains information on the causes of back pain and a chart on which treatments are "beneficial," "unlikely to be beneficial," and "unknown," but the site is sponsored by various companies, including drug companies, which stand to profit from the information.

Others example are www.lbackpain.com, a purely commercial site sponsored by chiropractors. They will be happy to sell you mattresses, back supports, traction devices, hot packs, and so forth. www.badback.com is an Australian supplier of braces, lumbar supports, pillows, creams, gels, and so on.

Looking at PubMed

PubMed is the Internet site of the National Institutes of Health (NIH), our government agency responsible for health issues. PubMed contains scientific medical articles. Doctors use this site to find the latest published research articles on any given health topic. Although this is an excellent resource for health professionals, the medical and scientific articles are difficult for the average person to understand. There are about a thousand scientific articles published each year related to back pain. If you are particularly motivated to find the latest information and to wade through the medical and scientific nature of these articles, you can find this website at www. ncbi.nlm.nih.gov/entrez/query.

10

Face-to-Face with Your Family Physician

If you've tried the simple solutions in Chapter 8 and your back pain has not gone away within six to eight weeks, you need to see your family physician or primary care doctor, a generalist trained in handling a variety of medical problems. The main reason is to find out exactly why you are hurting.

Don't skip this step by making an appointment with a spine specialist or orthopedic surgeon. As you've seen, back pain has many different causes, many of them only indirectly related to the spine. Your own problem may involve your kidneys or even your circulatory system, which is why your next step should be a visit to your regular doctor.

Depending on what your physician finds, he or she may or may not refer you to a specialist. (By the way, if you do need a specialist, your doctor is duty-bound by a professional code of ethics to refer you to one, regardless of what your insurance company or HMO would prefer.)

▮ What to Expect During the Examination

When you visit your doctor, be sure to explain all of the following:

- When the trouble started
- If you had a fall or injury within two days before the trouble started
- Exactly where and when you hurt, in detail
- How it feels (again, in detail)
- How the problem affects your daily life
- What medicines you've taken for it (both over-the-counter drugs such as Tylenol and prescription medications)
- Any other drugs you may be using (including drugs for other illnesses or conditions, as well as any recreational drugs)
- What other things you've tried (heat, cold, bed rest, walking, yoga, etc.)

Your doctor knows your own medical history better than anyone else (except maybe you), so he or she is in the very best position to help you. Since many different kinds of medical problems can cause back pain, your doctor can put together the different pieces and make some very good guesses about what your problem is.

For this reason, don't hide or withhold any information from your doctor, especially any drugs (including illegal drugs) you might be taking. (We have never known a physician to violate the principle of patient confidentiality and inform the police of a patient's illegal drug use.)

After talking to you, your doctor will do a physical examination. You will need to get undressed so that the doctor can see your back and legs. The doctor will look at the following:

- The curvature of your spine (any abnormal curving is known as scoliosis or kyphosis)
- The flexibility or stiffness of your spine

- Areas that are tender or have muscle spasms
- How you walk
- How you get on and off the examining table

Your doctor will also test the reflexes in your knees and ankles and check the strength in your legs.

Depending on the history and physical examination, your doctor may order some X-rays and basic laboratory tests. These are called screening tests because the doctor wants to screen out some of the unlikely (but possible) ugly things such as infection and cancer. (These and other tests are described in Chapter 11.)

Ask your doctor exactly what tests are being ordered. Write these down and check them against the ones discussed in Chapter 11. At this point, complex, expensive tests such as CT scans, myelograms, and MRIs are usually not necessary, so if your doctor orders them, ask why. And, as always, if there's anything about the exam or tests that you don't understand or that you'd like explained, ask your doctor immediately.

Once the test results come back (in about two or three days), the doctor will let you know what they showed or didn't show. If the results are normal, that's a good thing, and you can relax a bit. You still won't have a specific diagnosis—or perhaps you'll be diagnosed with lower back strain, which is a valid but very general diagnosis. Either way, your chances for a full and relatively quick recovery are excellent. Your doctor will probably give you a prescription for a pain medicine (but *not* an addictive narcotic) and may send you to a physical therapist for treatment.

About 80% of the time, the therapy and the pain medication will be successful, and within a few weeks you can dispense with both and return to a normal life. (The back pain may come back sometime in the future, but if it does, you can simply visit your regular doctor again and, except in highly unusual cases, receive the same successful treatment.)

If your regular doctor does find a specific problem with your spine, such as scoliosis, a fracture, an infection, or a spondylolisthesis (a problem in which two vertebrae have begun to slip apart—see Chapter 2 for details), then physical therapy won't help. Your doctor will probably need to refer you to a specialist.

Another possibility is that your doctor will discover a problem in another organ that you're feeling as back pain. These problems most commonly involve the kidneys or, in women, the reproductive system. However, the pain may also be the result of abnormalities in certain blood vessels. All of these situations result in *referred* pain, because the problem itself is not in the spine, but it is being *felt* in the spine; that is, the body is referring the pain from one part of the body to another part. In this case, the affected organ or area will need treatment. Your regular doctor may be able to do this, or he or she may need to send you to a specialist.

▋ Do You Have the Right Physician?

We hope that you're fortunate enough to already have a regular doctor whom you like and trust. If so, you can skip this brief section.

But what if you don't have a regular doctor or your trusted physician is retiring or moving away? What if you've become unhappy with your current doctor? And what if you've been assigned to a stranger by your health plan? How do you know this is someone you can trust?

Let's review the attributes of a good physician. At a minimum, any good doctor will do the following:

- Schedule appointments within a reasonable time
- Listen to you carefully
- Ask you questions about your condition

- Examine you carefully
- Test your leg reflexes and muscle strength
- Order all necessary and appropriate tests
- Interpret the results of these tests for you

What you *don't* want is a doctor who asks you only a couple of brief questions; doesn't ask you to get fully undressed; doesn't do reflex testing in your legs; doesn't test your leg muscle strength; or doesn't order any lab tests or X-rays. And after such a cursory exam, if the doctor says it's all in your head, it is definitely time to find another doctor.

Similarly, if the doctor tells you that your problem is chronic back pain, then get out of his or her office and find someone else. This is not a diagnosis; all the doctor has done is put a name on what you already knew you had. You deserve a real diagnosis and correct treatment, not a restatement of the obvious.

There's nothing wrong with trying an unknown doctor or going to the person your HMO (health maintenance organization) assigns you to. But if the physician doesn't meet all the criteria described previously, contact your health plan ombudsperson and insist on seeing another doctor. (For details on getting fair treatment from HMOs and insurance companies, see Chapter 14.)

If you've got a list of physicians to choose from but you don't know a thing about any of them, talk to your friends, your coworkers, and members of your extended family. Ask these people if they trust and appreciate their own doctor. If a physician whom someone mentions gets high marks, get his or her name and phone number and give this doctor a try. Also ask for referrals from a psychologist, counselor, or massage therapist if you see any of these professionals.

■ The Bottom Line

We can't overstress the importance of having an excellent primary care doctor. Remember, you are interested in getting two things: (1) the right diagnosis and (2) the right treatment. But you can't get the right treatment if you've been given a wrong diagnosis. And the more trustworthy and skilled your regular doctor is, the better your chance that his or her diagnosis will be correct.

For example, consider Gary, an 18-year-old boy whom one of us (Dr. Winter) saw about twenty years ago. He had had lower back pain for about six months, and it was steadily getting worse. He went to a family practice physician who took X-rays, looked them over, and saw an abnormal area in Gary's third lumbar vertebra. The doctor diagnosed a benign (noncancerous) bone defect and told Gary not to worry because the problem would go away on its own.

But it didn't; in fact, the affected area got bigger and more painful. Gary told this to his doctor, who told him to give it more time and repeated that the problem would go away by itself.

When Gary came to me six months later, he was almost completely paralyzed. We did tests of our own and decided that surgery was needed. When my team did surgery, we found that Gary had a malignant tumor of the spine that was destroying bone and pressing on his spinal nerves.

After two major surgeries, radiation treatment, and chemotherapy, Gary recovered fully. However, if he had received the right diagnosis the first time, he would not have become paralyzed, and he would not have needed surgery at all. His regular doctor had failed to listen to his complaints about increasing pain and weakness.

Another example is Gloria, a 41-year-old schoolteacher whose problem was thoracic back pain (pain in the area behind the chest). Her chest X-rays were normal, yet she had suffered from this pain for several years, and it kept getting worse and worse. Eventually, she had to give up golf, her favorite sport.

Gloria showed some signs of depression, so her doctor told her that her problem was psychological and prescribed antidepressants. These did not help at all; neither did psychological counseling. Finally, after suffering for five years, she went to see an orthopedic specialist, who examined her and sent her to me. Gloria's MRI revealed that she had Scheuermann's disease in the thoracic spine, with several degenerated discs. I ordered discograms, which pinpointed the source of her pain. A spine fusion operation completely eliminated her pain, and she went back to golfing six months later.

And her depression? It completely disappeared. It turned out to be the *result* of her chronic pain, not the cause.

Spine centers around the country have thousands of these stories. And they're all the result of some doctor failing to make a correct diagnosis.

▍ Ensuring a Correct Diagnosis

What can *you* do to help ensure that your doctor arrives at the correct diagnosis (and thus the correct treatment)?

First, get a basic education about your spine and what can go wrong with it by reading this book and referring to it as often as necessary. Second, ask your doctor about anything you don't fully understand. If your doctor tells you that your problem is a herniated disc, ask for an explanation of exactly what that is, why it's a problem, and what can (and should) be done about it. If there are two or more possible courses of action, ask for details about each one, including the pros, cons, risks, cost, and rate of success for each.

What if your doctor says, "I really don't know what you have; let me send you to a specialist who has a lot of experience with backs"? Or, "Well, I'm not sure what you've got, but my best guess is this . . ."?

Believe it or not, these are *good* signs because they mean you're in the hands of an honest doctor. Remember, for the most part, medicine is as much art as science, which is why doctors give you their best medical *opinions*. Sometimes the evidence will point very clearly to one particular cause, but in other cases there might be some ambiguity, several possible causes, or conflicting symptoms. In the face of uncertainty, a good physician will explain the nature of the uncertainty and either order more tests, send you to a specialist, or give you a list of potential next steps from which to choose. Chapter 12 provides guidance in finding specialists.

▌ The Physical Therapy Connection

If you're referred to a physical therapist, tell your doctor that you want to see a PT who understands the spine and has a lot of experience with it. *This is extremely important.* Don't go to a therapist who works mostly with stroke or heart attack victims. (If you're looking for a chef to cater an Italian banquet, would you hire a specialist in Chinese cuisine?) Only a PT with spine-related experience is fully qualified to design the ideal physical therapy program for you and your back. If your doctor says that she refers everyone to this PT or that your health plan requires her to refer you to a certain PT, don't just acquiesce. Remember, your health is at stake here. Find out exactly how much spine experience the PT has; if the doctor isn't sure, call the PT directly and ask. If the answer is questionable, push your doctor or your health plan ombudsperson to refer you to someone who has the necessary experience.

If you do get sent to physical therapy and you still hurt as much or more after six weeks, your problem could be something serious. Don't procrastinate. Call your doctor promptly and insist on a referral to a physician who specializes in the spine and who has had lots of experience treating it. If your doctor is unwilling to make this referral, talk to the ombudsperson at your HMO or health plan. Don't let yourself be given the runaround. Your health—and possibly your life—could depend on seeing the right specialist.

▌Second Opinions

This chapter should give you everything you need to find a talented and trustworthy family practice doctor; to help that doctor make the most accurate diagnosis; and to enable him or her to point you toward the right treatment and the quickest complete recovery. If for any reason you feel uncomfortable with or have doubts about a diagnosis, you should get a second medical opinion.

Contrary to popular belief, most doctors—indeed, all good physicians—are quite happy when their patients get a second opinion. After all, their primary concern is your health and well-being. If a second opinion confirms their own, then everyone can feel more confident about the appropriate course of treatment. And if the second opinion differs from their own, then it may have uncovered something important. This is, of course, a very good thing.

Never be afraid to get a second medical opinion because you're worried about hurting a doctor's feelings or harming your relationship with a doctor. In fact, if a doctor's ego is so fragile that getting a second opinion offends him or her, then you *definitely* need to find another doctor.

Your health plan may be another matter, however. If you feel a second opinion is warranted, talk to your health plan ombudsperson and explain the situation. Say why you're concerned that the diagnosis may not be accurate. Also explain that getting a second opinion will cost the health plan much less money than an inappropriate treatment.

This strategy will work occasionally. However, don't be surprised if in the end you have to pay for this second opinion yourself. Nevertheless, if you feel a second opinion is warranted, it is money well spent. If the second diagnosis agrees with the first, you will have bought yourself additional peace of mind; if it differs, you just may have saved your own life.

11

Tests

Although your doctors will find out a lot about you by listening to your history and doing a physical examination, they will probably need more help in finding out exactly what is wrong with your back. The human body is very complex, and pinpointing the exact cause of your back pain is vital. Fortunately, doctors have a host of tests available to help them understand the exact nature of back problems.

■ Laboratory Tests

Lab tests are done in a medical laboratory. The medical laboratory may be a part of a hospital, part of your doctor's clinic, or independent. Your doctor will order a lab test. A sample of your blood and/or urine will then be taken and sent to the lab. Your doctor will receive the results and use them to help understand your problem. The results of lab tests will typically be communicated to you at your next office visit or over the phone. Standard lab tests for patients with back problems include

- *Blood Count:* This simple test counts the red blood cells and the white blood cells. A healthy person has a normal range of red and white blood cells. If the number of either red or white blood cells falls out of the normal range, there is a problem. An increase in the number of white blood cells can indicate there is an infection in your body. A low red cell count means you are anemic and perhaps something is wrong with your bone marrow, which produces the red blood cells, or you are losing blood somewhere.

- *Sedimentation rate:* This blood test is used to determine if you have an infection or an inflammatory arthritis problem.

- *C-reactive protein:* This is another test helpful in diagnosing inflammatory arthritis or infection problems.

- *Serum protein analysis:* This blood test is most often used to diagnose multiple myeloma, a cancer of the bone marrow.

Exactly which tests are ordered depends on what the doctor has detected from your physical examination and history.

▌ X-Rays and Other Imaging

X-rays and other imaging studies produce films or pictures of your body that your doctors study to determine if any abnormalities are present. Once again, the particular studies ordered depend on what your doctors have detected on the history and physical examination. There is no single protocol for back problems.

Routine X-rays are often done in your doctor's office or clinic, although they can be done in the X-ray department of a hospital or at a stand-alone radiology center. X-rays produce an image of your bones. Your doctor will look at the X-ray to see if there is anything wrong or unusual with the bones in your back. You will likely have an X-ray taken from the front (with you standing to face the X-ray machine or lying on your back on the X-ray table) and from the side (with you lying down or standing up with your side facing the X-ray machine). Oblique X-rays are taken halfway between the front and side of your body. They add detail not seen on the routine front and side views. Spot films are very detailed X-rays that concentrate on just two or three vertebrae in your back. They are taken with you lying down. X-rays do not hurt, but they do use radiation. A typical spine X-ray requires about as much radiation as you would get from lying on a beach for three hours. X-rays should be avoided if you are pregnant.

Magnetic resonance imaging (MRI) is a common test for back problems. It does not use X-rays, so there is no radiation exposure. Rather, MRI uses a very powerful magnet to create and then read electrical energy in your body. The electrical energy is stored as digital information that is seen on a monitor or printed like an X-ray.

MRI requires that you lie very still for about fifteen to thirty minutes. It is performed in a tube-like structure, which can be difficult if you get claustrophobic in small or tight spaces. Some sedation may be necessary. So-called open-sided MRI units are available, but the quality of the images of the spine is much poorer than a regular MRI.

MRI is used by your doctor to detect many different spinal problems, especially disc disease, disc herniations, spinal stenosis, foraminal stenosis, spinal bone or disc infection, spondylolysis, and spinal cord or spinal bone tumors. MRI has dramatically changed the ability of doctors to diagnose the cause of back problems and to monitor the progress of treatment. There are no known risks of MRI except for those who have small pieces of metal in their body, which may be moved by the strong magnet. MRIs are done in the radiology department of a hospital or at an independent radiology center.

There is no contraindication to MRI with one exception. Small pieces of ferrous (iron-containing) metal can be moved by the powerful magnet so that, for example, a small flake of such metal in or near the eyeball can damage the eye. Pacemakers are another contraindication as well as some kinds of vascular stents. Large pieces of metal such as a total hip or spinal implants are NOT contraindications. Stainless steel spinal implants can interfere with getting a good image on the MRI, but titanium implants do not have that problem.

Computed axial tomography (**CT** or **CAT scan**) uses a large, complicated machine to create a very complex type of X-ray. The machine essentially takes pictures of a "slice" of your body, allowing your doctor to take a detailed look at any structure, especially the bones.

CT scans are done with the patient lying down. They take from fifteen to thirty minutes. The side effects or risks are those related to radiation. A CT scan requires more radiation than a plain X-ray. CT scans are done at either a radiology center or in the imaging (X-ray) department of a hospital.

A **bone scan** detects specific problems in the bones. A radioactive material is injected into the body and allowed to circulate for an hour or two. Then the patient is put under a Geiger counter (radiation detection device) to see if any area of the body "lights up" (as it would if the radioactive material has concentrated itself in one place). An infection or tumor in the back will light up a bone scan. Bone scans are sometimes used to detect spondylolysis (see Chapter 2). A bone scan uses only a very tiny amount of radiation, which is quickly eliminated from the body.

A **myelogram** is an X-ray test used to outline the nerves and spinal cord inside the spinal canal. A needle is placed into the spinal canal while the patient is under local anesthesia (the area where the doctor is working is numb). The needle is used to inject a water-soluble dye into the spinal canal. This dye outlines the nerves and spinal cord so that a detailed X-ray of the area can be obtained. The dye is gradually absorbed by the body and secreted in the urine. This used to be the standard test for the diagnosis of disc herniations, but it has almost been completely supplanted by the MRI scan. It is still useful for the diagnosis of spinal stenosis. It is also used extensively in evaluating the spinal canal in patients who have had a spine fusion with instrumentation, since the metal of the instrumentation interferes with getting a decent MRI image. This is done by a radiologist in a radiology unit of a hospital or in an independent radiology center.

A **CT myelogram** combines a myelogram with a CT scan. Dye is injected into the spinal canal, then a CT scan is done. This provides greater detail than either the myelogram or the CT scan done alone.

A **discogram** is an X-ray test used to diagnose disc problems. The doctor inserts a needle into the center of the disc. This is done with local anesthesia, since it is very important that the patient be awake and able to communicate with the doctor. The needle is used to inject sterile saline (salt) water into the disc in order to test the amount of pressure in the disc. This is followed by the injection of a radiopaque dye into the center of the disc. X-rays are taken to see the character of the disc, and sometimes CT scans are also taken to get an even better look. The doctor is also interested in the amount of pain or discomfort the patient has at the time of the injection.

This procedure is typically performed in a radiology suite of a hospital or independent radiology center. It is usually done by a radiologist, but sometimes a surgeon or pain management specialist administers the test.

▌Electrodiagnostic Tests

Electrodiagnostic tests use a gentle electric current to test how well the nerves are working.

An **electromyogram (EMG)** tests how well your nerves are able to control (or contract) your muscles. The nerves send impulses to your muscles to tell them when to work and when to rest. If a nerve is damaged or irritated, it cannot send impulses to the muscles like it used to.

Very thin needles are placed in certain muscles to record the electrical activity in them. This electrical activity is created by the nerves that run to those muscles. If there is no nerve supply or if the nerve supply is altered, the electrical activity in the muscles will not be normal. An EMG is used to test for irritated nerves or nerves that are not functioning normally. This test is usually done by neurologists or physical medicine and rehabilitation doctors. There are no risks.

Nerve conduction tests also detect nerve problems. Electrical impulses are sent through the nerves, and the speed at which these impulses travel is measured. If a nerve is damaged or irritated, it will conduct these impulses at a slower rate than normal.

▌ Block Tests

A **nerve root block** tests the health of the nerves where they exit the spine. Your doctor might order this test if you have a back problem that causes nerve pain in your legs. This test helps the doctor find out if a nerve is being pinched.

A needle is placed (under X-ray control) near the opening (the foramen) where the nerve root leaves the spine. The nerve is then injected with local anesthetic to numb it. If the pain in your leg goes away, then the doctor has found the nerve that is pinched and is causing your leg pain. This test is also used by spine surgeons to determine which nerve is the problem and exactly where to operate. It is usually done by a radiologist.

A **facet block** is used to find out if back pain is coming from one of the little joints in the spine called a facet joint. The doctor inserts a needle into the facet joint area and numbs the area with a local anesthetic. This information helps the doctor determine whether the injected facet joint is the problem.

12

Step-by-Step: Using the Back Care Pyramid

The Back Care Pyramid is your guide through the dizzying array of back care options. It is set up logically. The pyramid starts with the easiest and least expensive treatments. For most people with back problems—fully 98%—the first two levels, self-care and the care of their primary care doctor, are all that is needed to alleviate back pain. For those who need it, each ascending level is the next reasonable step in back care.

The Back Care Pyramid is built on the solid foundation of evidence-based medicine. At each step, the physician you see is committed to treatment that has stood the test of scientific rigor. Real evidence exists to show this treatment works. Evidence-based medicine is the clearest and straightest path from a place of back pain and disability to a place of healing.

At each ascending level of the pyramid, you will encounter physicians who are more and more specialized in treating the spine. You do not need to "hit" every step. It is perfectly fine to jump levels. For example, your primary care doctor may refer you directly to a spine surgeon if that is what you need.

The Back Care Pyramid

```
                    Spine
                   Surgeon

                Spine Specialist

            Orthopedic Surgeon
           Rehabilitation Physician

          Family/Primary Care Doctor

                  Self-Care
```

▌ Step 1: Self-Care

The Back Care Pyramid starts with the person with the most power to heal your back pain—you. With simple, inexpensive methods, such as stretching and lifestyle changes, most people can resolve their own back problem. Take the self-care step seriously. Give the recommendations outlined in Chapter 8 a serious go. If a diligent effort at self-care doesn't yield the results you were hoping for, it is time for step 2 of the Back Care Pyramid: a visit to your primary care doctor.

▌ Step 2: Your Primary Care Doctor

The first physician you will see face-to-face is your primary care doctor. The primary care doctor is a generalist trained in handling a variety of medical problems. Most primary care doctors are comfortable treating back pain, and they often act as advocates for their patients, coordinating their treatment programs.

Your primary care doctor's first order of business is twofold: (1) making certain there is nothing seriously wrong with your spine such as infection or cancer and (2) determining why you are hurting. He will arrive at a diagnosis by asking you questions, examining your back, and ordering tests if indicated. Upon arriving at a diagnosis, your primary care doctor will then begin appropriate treatment. This might include medications, education, and a referral to physical therapy.

Over the long haul, your primary care doctor will usually manage your case, referring you to different specialists as appropriate. Most primary care doctors have a network of specialists they know and trust. This network and the advocacy of your primary care doctor are invaluable in getting you to the right caregivers.

Your primary care doctor will be a family practice doctor or a general internist. Both types of doctors have completed medical school and residency. Family practice doctors specialize in general family care. Internists diagnose and medically treat (without surgery) disease in adults.

A physician-extender (someone who cares for patients under the supervision of a physician) such as a nurse practitioner (NP) or physician's assistant (PA) may serve as a primary care practitioner. Nurse practitioners are registered nurses with advanced training in a specialty such as adult or geriatric care. A master's degree is required for entry-level practice, and licensing is state regulated through the nursing board. The scope of practice for NPs varies from state to state (you can find this information by contacting the nursing board in your state). NPs perform many of the services done by doctors, often with an emphasis on nurturing and education and always under the supervision of a doctor.

A physician's assistant is a college graduate who has completed an accredited physician's assistant program that is approximately twenty-six months in length. PAs become licensed by passing a national certification exam. A PA is a representative of the physician, treating patients in a manner developed and directed by the supervising physician.

Your primary care doctor will likely treat you for six to eight weeks. After this length of time, if you are not better or if you are having new symptoms, the doctor may refer you to a specialist.

▋ Step 3: The Specialists

Specialists are physicians with advanced training in a specific area of medical care. The American Board of Medical Specialties recognizes twenty-four different types of specialists. The specialist you are most likely to see at this step of the Back Care Pyramid is an orthopedic surgeon or a rehabilitation doctor.

General Orthopedic Surgeon

An orthopedic surgeon or orthopedist specializes in the care of musculoskeletal system disorders (bones, joints, muscles, tendons, and ligaments). A general orthopedist will see a broad variety of orthopedic patients such as those with ankle sprains, knee strains, or back pain.

Because orthopedists have advanced training in musculoskeletal disorders, they offer more specialized care in diagnosing and treating back problems. They will confirm or refine the diagnosis you were given by your primary care doctor by conducting a history-taking interview, performing a clinical examination, and ordering further tests if indicated. Your orthopedist may prescribe medications, recommend a nonsurgical treatment, or refer you to a spine specialist or spine surgeon.

General Rehabilitation Medicine Doctor or Physiatrist

A rehabilitation doctor practices a medical specialty called physical medicine and rehabilitation (PM&R). Physiatrists utilize a wide variety of conservative treatments for musculoskeletal disorders, but they do not perform surgery. They typically treat the whole person, addressing physical, mental, and emotional issues. Your physiatrist will take your history, conduct a physical examination, and order diagnostic tests if indicated.

Physiatrists use medications, physical and therapeutic agents, exercise, and more to treat back pain. Your physiatrist may also refer you a physical therapist, occupational therapist, vocational rehabilitation specialist, or psychologist.

∎ Step 4: Spine Specialists

A spine specialist may be trained as an orthopedist, neurologist, or physiatrist. These doctors specialize in treating back problems, so the vast majority of their practice is dedicated to helping patients with back problems. Spine specialists typically have the most experience and thus the greatest diagnostic and treatment savvy for those with back problems.

Neurologist Spine Specialist

Neurologists specialize in the diagnosis and nonsurgical treatment of brain and nervous system disorders. They are trained to perform a thorough examination of all the important neurological (nerve-related) structures in the body. Neurologists often serve as consultants, especially in distinguishing a primary neurological problem from a musculoskeletal one. Neurologists are considered spine specialists if 80% or more of their practice consists of treating patients with back problems.

Orthopedic Spine Specialist

Orthopedists specializing in back problems are called orthopedic spine specialists. Their practice is almost solely dedicated to treating spine problems (usually 80% or more). Because they are so focused on caring for back problems, they know the latest in diagnosis and treatment. Orthopedic spine specialists make use of many types of treatments as well as the expertise of other doctors.

Physiatrist Spine Specialist

A physiatrist who focuses on treating back problems can be a spine specialist. In this case, 80% or more of the physiatrist's practice is focused on spine patients. The physiatrist who is a spine specialist offers many of the same types of treatment as a general physiatrist (such as physical and therapeutic modalities) but offers more specialized diagnostic and treatment knowledge and experience.

▌ Step 5: Spine Surgeons

Spine surgeons see the small minority of back pain patients who need surgery. They do 90% to 95% of their surgical work in the spine. When seeking a spine surgeon, a patient doesn't want the neurosurgeon who does mostly brain surgery or the orthopedic surgeon who does mostly hip and knee replacements. The spine surgeon's area of expertise should be clarified *before* making an appointment. Simply ask the person scheduling your appointment whether the surgeon does the majority of his surgical work in the spine. If that person cannot answer your question, ask for someone who can. Even if your primary care doctor referred you to the surgeon, still ask this question.

Spine Neurosurgeons

In general, neurosurgeons provide surgical care for disorders of the brain, spinal cord, and nervous system. Neurosurgeons who specialize in spine surgery have chosen to focus their practice on the surgical care of back problems. They tend to perform surgery for tumors of the spinal cord or nerve root, herniated discs, and spinal stenosis (decompression).

Orthopedic Spine Surgeons

Some doctors who are trained as orthopedic surgeons choose to focus their practice on the surgical care of back problems. These spine surgeons tend to perform surgery for herniated discs, scoliosis and kyphosis, disc degeneration (spinal fusion), and spinal stenosis (decompression).

Orthopedic spine surgeons and neurosurgical spine surgeons function at the two top levels of the Back Care Pyramid. Don't think you will automatically have surgery if you see a spine surgeon. These surgeons perform surgery on the minority of the patients they see. Spine surgeons are best qualified to determine if you need surgery. There is a danger in nonsurgeons not recognizing when surgery is appropriate. You are then left with inadequate treatment such as overuse of addicting narcotic pain medications.

■■

PHYSICIANS OF THE BACK CARE PYRAMID

Professional Title	Education and Training	Scope of Practice
Family Practice Doctor	Medical school, 3-year residency	Diagnosis and treatment of a wide variety of illnesses. First step in care of undiagnosed health concerns.
Internist	Medical school, 3-year residency	Trained to understand all major organ systems and treat a variety of illnesses.
General Orthopedic Surgeon	Medical school, 5-year residency	Surgical and nonsurgical treatment of a broad range of musculoskeletal disorders.
General Rehabilitation Physician	Medical school, 4-year residency	Diagnosis and treatment of both acute and chronic pain and musculoskeletal disorders.
Neurologist	Medical school, 4-year residency	Diagnosis and treatment of nervous system disorders.
Orthopedic Surgeon Spine Specialist	Medical school, 5-year residency	Focuses 90% or more of practice on treating spine problems.
Rehabilitation Physician Spine Specialist	Medical school, 4-year residency	Focuses 90% or more of practice on treating spine problems.
Neurosurgeon	Medical school, 5-year residency, spine fellowship	Trained in most types of spine surgery, especially those that are nerve related.
Orthopedic Surgeon	Medical school, 5-year residency, spine fellowship	Trained in most types of spine surgery, especially those related to the musculoskeletal system.

▮ Checking Out a Doctor's Credentials

Knowing a doctor's credentials and expertise can help you find the best physician for you. It can also help you know what kind of care you should expect.

Use the following questions as a guideline for important information. You can get some of this information when you schedule your appointment or from the office staff. Any remaining questions can be addressed directly to the doctor. But be realistic about how many questions to ask the physician. If you spend too much time asking questions about expertise, you shortchange the amount of time the doctor has to evaluate your condition.

1. What degree does the doctor hold?

Many professionals go by the title "doctor" even when they are not medical physicians. This group includes those with a PhD (in disciplines such as exercise physiology, nursing, physics, or history), chiropractors (DC means doctor of chiropractic), and those with "doctorates" in alternative medicine practice. The initials MD stand for medical doctor. You might also see the initials DO with your doctor's name. This stands for doctor of osteopathy. The education for DOs is the same as that for MDs. MDs and DOs have completed medical school and residency and work within the confines of standard medical practice. All the professionals within the Back Care Pyramid are medical doctors.

Chapter 3 discusses the training and background of practitioners such as chiropractors who provide alternative treatment. These professionals have training in their particular field, but they have not been to medical school and do not have a medical degree.

2. What is the doctor's specialty?

Use the Physicians of the Back Care Pyramid table on page 132 and the information outlined earlier in this chapter to understand the differences between the specialists in the Back Care Pyramid. If you know the scope of practice and typical treatments offered for back pain by each specialist, you will have a better idea what to expect from that doctor.

3. What is the doctor's hospital affiliation?

Ideally your doctor is affiliated with a reputable, well-equipped hospital. If the doctor is a staff member or attending physician at a given hospital, he or she has admitting privileges. This may become important to you if you need to be hospitalized or have surgery.

4. Is the doctor covered by your insurance plan?

Your choice of doctors may be limited to those in your health plan (unless you are willing to pay out of pocket). Check your health plan directory to find a list of eligible doctors, or call the doctor's office to see if he or she is part of your health plan network.

Asking about Experience

A doctor's credentials tell you about his or her general competence. They indicate that the doctor has the right education and training. Beyond credentials, the best doctors also have depth of experience. Research shows that doctors who have a lot of experience with a condition tend to have better success treating it. For example, the American College of Surgeons advises open heart surgery patients to look for a surgeon who performs at least 150 such procedures a year. When it comes to complicated medical problems and procedures, practice makes perfect.

Questions you might ask include: How often do you see patients with my type of back problem? What treatment did you use to help them? If a certain procedure such as surgery is recommended, ask: How many times have you performed this particular procedure? What is your success rate with this procedure? What sort of complications have you experienced with this procedure? How often do complications occur and how are they managed?

■ The All-Important Bedside Manner

A doctor's interpersonal skill and ability to communicate are very important. Expect your doctor to treat you like a partner in your own health care. Test results, medications, and procedures should be explained in a thorough, understandable manner. Your questions should be answered carefully and respectfully. Finding the right doctor often comes down to a gut reaction, knowing intuitively that he or she fits the bill. The following tips can help you come to a good conclusion:

- The doctor's office staff should be considerate and helpful.
- The doctor should focus on you during the consultation without interruptions by other staff or by phone calls (unless it is an emergency).
- You should not feel rushed through the visit.
- The physician should listen to you.
- The doctor should treat you like a capable person.
- Thorough and clear explanations should be given for medical procedures and test results.
- You should be given a chance to ask questions.
- You should feel comfortable.
- You should be encouraged to call if questions arise concerning your treatment.

Sometimes it makes sense to give the relationship between you and your doctor time to develop. It takes more than one visit to get to know each other.

13

Choosing the Right Treatment

You may be reading this chapter because you woke up yesterday with a miserable backache after helping your brother move a lot of furniture the day before. Or you might have a backache that's been bugging you for a month, and the over-the-counter pain pills and a heating pad just haven't helped. Or you might have back problems that have been persistent for over a year even though you've seen three different doctors.

These three situations are quite different. The first situation is an acute problem, the second, a subacute problem, and the third, a chronic problem. We have emphasized these differences because the treatment for each situation is quite different.

The most important thing is that good treatment depends on good diagnosis. *Back pain is not a diagnosis; it is just a symptom.* It is no different from a headache—a symptom that can be caused by a huge number of problems ranging from anxiety to a brain tumor.

▮ Acute Back Pain

Acute back pain is something you've had for only a few days. It may or may not be related to an injury at home or at work. Most of the time, the treatment you choose will be simple, inexpensive, and not require you to see a doctor.

Read Chapter 1 again. Eighty percent of acute back pain problems go away in a few days. You can help yourself with over-the-counter (nonprescription) medications such as aspirin, ibuprofen, or acetaminophen, heat or ice packs, and resting in the contour position (but no more than two or three days of bed rest). You are functioning at the lowest level of the Back Care Pyramid.

There are a few warning signs that should lead you to call your doctor right away if you experience them: back pain with fever, back pain with strong leg pain, back pain with weakness or numbness in one or both legs, and back pain with loss of control of your bladder or bowels. Pain worse at night is also a danger sign. You will probably go to the emergency room and be seen by a spine specialist. In these rare circumstances, you jump to the highest two levels of the pyramid.

▮ Subacute Back Pain

Subacute back pain is pain that is still around after a month or so. As we said before, 80% of acute back pain goes away in about a week, but 20% doesn't.

If your pain continues, it's time to move up the Back Care Pyramid and see your family doctor or primary care doctor, the second level of the pyramid. At this point, you really need to know why you are having back pain. Since good treatment depends on good diagnosis, now is the time to try to find that diagnosis.

When you see the doctor, you will have your history taken, a physical examination, perhaps some basic X-rays, and possibly some basic lab tests. About 80% of the time, these tests will not provide a specific diagnosis, but more importantly they will show whether you have specific abnormalities that need special treatment.

If you are without a specific diagnosis at this point, you need to get treatment appropriate for your situation. What should you choose? You will discuss the options with your doctor. The two most common treatments are physical therapy and chiropractic. For subacute back pain in the absence of a specific diagnosis (non-specific back pain), both have proven valuable in clinical trials (evidence-based medicine), with physical therapy holding a slight edge in benefit. Details about these two treatments can be found in Chapter 3. With five or six treatments, about 80% of subacute back pain patients will experience significant improvement. Although recurrences are common, these can easily be dealt with.

▌ Chronic Back Pain

What do you do if you are in the 20% who do not respond to this treatment? You should go back to your family doctor or primary care doctor and get his or her advice. Almost always this means moving up the Back Care Pyramid to a specialist. There are several medical specialties dealing with back pain including orthopedic surgery, neurosurgery, physical medicine and rehabilitation, and neurology. Your family doctor will help you find a good specialist (see Chapter 16).

This move up the Back Care Pyramid will involve having your history taken again, a more detailed physical examination, and more tests. It is at this point that CT scans and/or MRI scans may be ordered.

The specialist's recommendations depend on what he or she finds on the examination and tests. About 80% of patients can get a specific diagnosis. Once this diagnosis has been made, the treatment choices become more obvious.

Let us say, for example, that your problem has been diagnosed as an isthmic spondylolisthesis of L_5 with degenerative disc disease at L_5-S_1. The isthmic spondylolisthesis of L_5 was diagnosed on plain X-rays, but it was not until you got the MRI that the disc degeneration became known.

Does this mean you have to have surgery? No, not at all. In fact, most patients with this problem get along well without surgery, but they may need an intense physical therapy program different from a generic therapy program, or perhaps a brace and therapy. Chiropractic care does not treat this problem well.

The specialist can discuss with you the various alternatives including surgery, bracing, physical therapy, and medications. Medications alone are not the answer, since you have a specific organic problem causing the pain, and pain medications only cover up the pain rather than get at the cause of it.

If you are still miserable after trying the therapy, you need to take another step up the pyramid. If you have a degenerated disc at L_5-S_1 with an isthmic spondylolisthesis at L_5, you will go to a spine surgeon, since it is a surgically treatable problem.

If you see the surgeon and surgery is recommended, do you immediately choose it? No, you need to listen to the details of the surgery, the possible risks and complications, and if in doubt, get a second opinion. Then and only then do you choose which path to take. You either have to have the surgery to decrease the pain, choose to live with the pain, or go to a pain management specialist who will put you on long-term narcotics or refer you to get an implanted spinal cord stimulator or morphine pump.

What if you see a spine specialist and there is no surgically treatable problem? The answer lies in why you are having the pain and again underlines the need to get a diagnosis.

If you are found to have ankylosing spondylitis, a rheumatologic problem that involves the spine, the treatment is medical with special drugs prescribed by a rheumatologist.

If you have an infection in the spine, 90% of the time the treatment is antibiotics alone, but surgery is necessary in 10% of patients. Do you get to choose which path? Not really, since there are very specific indications for each one. The surgeon will discuss them with you; that is, you participate in the decision, but the final choice is based on the medical indications.

14

Dealing with Your Health Insurance

The financial dimensions of medical care are complex and rarely consumer-friendly. Yet there are five critical steps you can take toward getting the back care you want without breaking your personal bank.

Getting the Most from Health Insurance Benefits

1. Remember the three key principles of health insurance (see page 143).
2. Answer specific questions about what your policy covers and what it does not cover.
3. Before you get treatment, contact the payer.
4. Keep detailed records of your contacts with treatment providers and health insurers.
5. Learn about the three stages in resolving conflict with a payer.

▮ Step 1: Remember the three key principles of health insurance

Medical care is not free. Someone must pay for it. The only question is who the financially responsible party—also called the *payer*—will be. If not a government agency such as Medicare, the payer is a private health insurance company.

You might assume that private health insurance companies are in the business of being payers—that is, paying claims to cover the costs of medical treatment. That's logical but inaccurate. The first principle of health insurance is that *insurers are in business to make a profit, not to pay claims.* Paying claims for medical treatment decreases profits. If an insurance company can find a legal reason not to pay a claim, then it will not pay.

This may sound like a cynical statement. It is not meant that way. Rather, this principle simply describes the way that health care finances work. Also remember that insurance companies are not unique in their attitude toward making payments. Fundamentally, no one really wants to pay out money unless they have to. That's true for individuals as well as organizations, nonprofit or for-profit, of any size.

A second key principle is that the core of your relationship with a health insurer is a legal contract, also called a *policy*. This contract spells out what treatments the insurer will pay for, how much and when it will pay, and what treatments it will not pay for.

When it comes to contracts, knowledge is power, which leads to a third principle: Be sure to find out what rights are granted to you in your health insurance contract and what responsibilities you are required to meet. It's up to you to understand the contract and use its provisions to your benefit. *Failure to meet your payer's requirements could mean that you have to cover the cost of some or all of your medical care.*

The fact that health insurers want to make a profit is reflected in their contract with you. You'll want to find out what specific medical treatments are covered in your contract and whether they're covered fully or partially. However, it's equally important to find out what treatments are *not* covered and what to do when you believe a specific treatment is covered under your contract and your insurer disagrees.

You do not have to become an expert in health insurance. Rather, your task is to understand the key elements of your contract and find out how they apply to you, especially to treatments for your back.

Principle 1
Insurers are in business to make a profit, not to pay claims.

Principle 2
The core of your relationship with an insurer is a legal contract—your policy.

Principle 3
It's up to you to understand your policy, and failure to do this can cost you money.

▌Step 2: Answer specific questions about what your policy covers and what it does not cover

Perhaps you're in a position right now to choose your health insurance through an employer, union, or professional association. If so, take time to choose the best policy you can afford, remembering that "best" is in the eye of the beholder. The best policy for someone else may not be the best for you. It all depends on what you value most.

Some people want low premiums above all. Other people want a policy that covers specific treatments even if this means paying a higher premium.

- Ask for plan summaries and sales literature about the policies that you're considering.
- When you find a policy that interests you, go beyond the summaries and read the actual contract (which is the legally binding document).
- Ask your insurance agent or employee benefits representative to explain any part of the contract that confuses you.
- Find out if there's a period of time after you first sign up for a policy (often thirty days) during which you can change your mind, go back to the drawing board, and select another policy.

You might be able to get an independent rating of the health insurance policy you're considering. For example, the National Committee for Quality Assurance (NCQA) maintains a website where you can enter policy information and get "report cards" for various plans. Access this site at www.ncqa.org.

However, it's far more likely that you must simply live with a health insurance plan that you already have. Your job at this point is to "diagnose" your health insurance—to dig into your current coverage, study the fine print, take full advantage of the coverage you have, and spot potential problems. This might sound like a lot of work, but it's worth the effort. *Perhaps the most effective way to prevent health insurance hassles is to know up front what is and is not covered by your policy.* Gaining this knowledge now, before you make major treatment decisions or enter into a dispute with your health insurer, can prevent needless aggravation and surprise expenses.

Taking time to understand your policy can help you avoid situations such as these:

- You go to see a spine specialist who is not authorized to provide treatment under your health plan and wind up with a large bill to pay out of your own pocket.

- You go to a specialist who *is* authorized to provide treatment, but you decide to get a second opinion from another specialist. Later, you find out that the second specialist is *not* authorized under your plan. Again, you end up with an unexpected bill.
- You get authorization in advance to get a second opinion and find out that the physician authorized to give this opinion has no expertise on your condition.

It is beyond the scope of this chapter to give you detailed scenarios for dealing with such situations. The most appropriate actions for you to take will depend on coverage provided by your health insurance policy. And policies differ greatly. However, the steps presented in this chapter can give you a process for *choosing* which actions to take, no matter what kind of policy you have.

A key theme in this book is the idea of taking control of all areas of your back care. See, for example, the suggestions for choosing treatments listed in Chapter 13 and the instructions for taking control when you need surgery in Chapter 17. When it comes to health insurance, taking control starts with answering the following questions about your coverage.

Do I have an indemnity policy or a managed care policy?

Just a few decades ago, the standard health insurance policy for most Americans was an indemnity, or fee-for-service, plan. Such plans typically offer these features:

- You get medical treatment from just about any physician or hospital that you choose.
- When you get treatment, you pay a certain amount (called a deductible) out of your own pocket.
- After you pay the deductible, your health care provider sends a bill for medical treatment to your insurer.

- The insurer pays 80% of the usual and customary charges for the treatment. You pay the remaining 20%.

This kind of plan still exists, but it is no longer the norm. Instead, many Americans get their health insurance through managed care companies. These companies use various strategies to control health care costs.

Managed care comes under various names including health maintenance organizations (HMOs), preferred provider organizations (PPOs), and point-of-service (POS) plans. Whatever their name, such companies contract with a network of physicians, hospitals, and other professionals who agree to provide health care at a discount. In return:

- You rarely see any paperwork, including bills, for the treatment you receive.
- You pay a single premium that pays for all or most of your medical care.
- Your policy usually covers a greater range of treatments than an indemnity plan.
- Your choice of health care providers is limited to professionals who belong to the network.

Currently, many health insurance policies blend features of indemnity plans and managed care plans. For example, you might belong to an HMO that allows you to see health care providers outside the network as long as you agree to accept indemnity coverage for these providers. While such hybrid policies give consumers more options, they involve increasingly complex policies. It's now more important than ever before that you thoroughly understand what you're buying.

What treatments are included or excluded?

When you read a health insurance policy, pay special attention to sections with titles such as *policy benefits* and *exclusions* or *limita-*

tions on coverage. Here is where you'll find lists of treatments that are covered and those that are not covered.

Think about the kind of treatments you want to get for your back condition and find out if your policy will cover them. In general, treatments by physicians and by professionals who receive referrals *from* physicians are the most likely to be covered. Many policies include coverage for physical therapy and chiropractic care. However, complementary and alternative treatments, such as services from acupuncturists and massage therapists, are often *not* covered.

Be sure to read your policy for two special categories of treatment. The first is *experimental treatments*. These are the latest medications, surgeries, and other procedures for a specific condition. Do not assume that your health insurance will cover them. Insurers may even balk at covering treatments approved by the U.S. Food and Drug Administration (FDA). An example is the artificial disc approved in October 2004 as a treatment for lower back pain, which at this writing is not widely insured. Health insurers generally wait until a treatment has a substantial track record and a predictable cost before taking it off the "experimental" list.

Also check the definitions for *elective treatments*. The word *elective* means "optional" in the eyes of the insurer. For example, some types of spine surgery are considered elective even though they could benefit people whose back condition involves disabling levels of pain.

To what extent can I choose my health care providers?

Some indemnity policies allow you to choose any physician who you want to see. If your health insurance comes from a managed care organization, however, you'll be restricted to a list of approved physicians and other health care providers. From this list, you'll choose a primary care physician who will coordinate your care and refer you to specialists.

If you're switching health insurance plans and your current primary care physician is not on the list, you'll need to find a new one. Some consumers find this troubling, especially when they've spent years seeing a physician who has treated their back condition successfully.

Inspect the provider list included with your health plan. Determine whether any physicians or other providers who you especially want to see are included. Perhaps you can persuade your primary physician to refer you to an outside provider; that is, one who's not on the list. But remember: *If you don't get a referral or other prior authorization from your health insurer, you might have to pay the total rather than partial or copay costs of such a provider.*

As you read your health insurance policy, look for answers to these specific questions:

- Do you need a referral from your primary care physician in order to see a specialist such as a spine surgeon?
- Are there restrictions or limitations on where you must go for nonsurgical treatments such as injections and physical therapy?
- Are there restrictions or limitations on where you must go for diagnostic tests such as MRIs and discograms?
- Which hospitals are you allowed to use?
- Where are you allowed to go for after-hours and emergency care?
- Are the approved providers and hospitals located in places that are convenient for you?
- If you need medical care while away from home, do you need to get an authorization from the insurer first?
- If you get a referral to a specialist who is authorized under your insurance, are you limited in the number of visits you can make to this specialist? If you want more visits, can you request them yourself or do you need to see your primary care physician first?

What costs will I have to pay?

Few if any health insurance plans will cover all the costs of your health care. Some policies cover more than others, but there will always be times when you'll need to reach into your own pocket. Costs to you generally include

- A health insurance premium, which is often due every month
- Deductibles
- Copayments for office visits, diagnostic tests, surgeries, and hospital stays
- Out-of-pocket expenses for health providers outside an approved network

It's difficult to predict how much you will spend on health care. Yet it's useful to estimate your total costs, especially if you're comparing health insurance policies. List the treatments you plan to get over the coming year, and estimate how much you'll pay under each policy you're considering. Find out if any premium discounts will apply to you if you don't smoke or if you engage in other activities that may prevent health problems. Subtract those discounts from your total costs.

Also think about possible costs beyond the coming year. Look for any limits the policy imposes on treatments for a major long-term illness. Some health insurers place limits on the treatments they will cover each year or over the entire life of the policy.

Who will pay for a covered treatment if I have duplicate benefits?

Don't expect to make money on health insurance. You might have more than one source of health insurance such as a policy through your employer and another through your spouse's employer. Even so, you won't receive double payment for a covered treatment.

Insurers will coordinate their benefits so that they never pay more than 100% of any treatment cost. Look for a section of your policy titled *coordination of benefits* to find out how this is done and what you're required to do when it applies.

Do I have Medicare coverage, Medicaid coverage, or both?

Title XVIII of the Social Security Act—originally called Health Insurance for the Aged and Disabled—is now commonly known as Medicare. This legislation set up a health insurance program for older Americans to complement the retirement, survivors, and disability insurance benefits under earlier laws.

You may hear people talk about Part A and Part B when referring to Medicare. These terms refer to two different kinds of coverage: Part A offers hospital insurance, and Part B offers medical insurance for certain treatments provided outside a hospital. Part A is generally automatic and free to people age 65 or older who are eligible for Social Security or Railroad Retirement benefits. Part B is available for a monthly premium.

A third element of Medicare known as Part C or Medicare+ Choice is the Medicare Advantage program. This program provides options to get additional health care benefits from insurers in the private sector.

The newest element of Medicare is a prescription drug benefit implemented in 2006 known as Part D. This is a complex and confusing program. Part D requires a highly variable monthly premium, though it offers subsidies to hold down costs for people who qualify for the coverage.

Many people who are covered by Medicare are also covered by another health insurance plan. If a specific medical treatment is covered by both Medicare and the other plan, then a policy called Medicare Secondary Payer (MSP) decides which will pay first. Remember that when it comes to making this decision, federal law takes precedence over state law and the provisions of health insurance policies.

If you have Medicare coverage, the Centers for Medicare and Medicaid Service suggest that you take the following actions to make sure your claims for medical treatment are correctly paid:

- Respond promptly to questionnaires and letters sent by MSP.
- Remember that changes in employment or health insurance companies may affect your claims payment. Contact the coordination of benefits contractor for Medicare about such changes.
- Also contact the coordination of benefits contractor if you are involved in an automobile accident, a workers' compensation case, or legal action on your behalf for a medical claim.

A coordination of benefits contractor for Medicare can give you more details. You have the right to appeal any decision about your Medicare coverage. Look for a list of your appeal rights on the back of the Explanation of Medicare Benefits or Medicare Summary Notice sent by Medicare. Medicare is required to tell you why it decided to deny payment for a medical treatment and what steps you can take to appeal the decision.

Medicaid is another piece of federal legislation—one that's specifically designed to provide health insurance for people with a low income. Even though it is a national program, each state makes its own decisions about who qualifies for the program, what kind of treatments are covered, and what deductibles or copayments apply. A person who qualifies for Medicaid in one state might not qualify in another state. And states can change their Medicaid policies from year to year.

Sometimes a treatment is covered under both Medicare and Medicaid. When this happens, Medicare pays first. Medicaid is always the payer of last resort.

Seven Questions to Ask about Your Health Insurance Policy

1. Do I have an indemnity policy or a managed care policy?
2. What treatments are included or excluded?
3. To what extent can I choose my health care providers?
4. What costs will I have to pay?
5. Who will pay for a covered treatment if I have duplicate benefits?
6. Do I have Medicare coverage, Medicaid coverage, or both?
7. Whom do I contact with questions about my policy?

Whom do I contact with questions about my policy?

The ID card for your health insurance probably includes a phone number and other contact information for a customer service representative or members services office. This is usually the first place to call when you have a complaint or questions about which providers you can see, what treatments are covered, how much you have to pay for treatments, and similar issues.

You might also get answers from your employee benefits manager if you receive health insurance through your job. Keep this person's phone number on hand as well.

Don't be afraid to call these numbers. Do so whenever you get a bill, referral, or any other communication from your health insurer that you do not understand. When in doubt, ask for clarification, no matter how insignificant the matter seems.

▌ Step 3: Before you get treatment, contact the payer

When it comes to treatments for back problems or other conditions, no one likes surprises. Surprises that cost you money are the least desirable of all. Once you have read through your insurance policy and answered the questions listed in step 3, contact the payer that you think is responsible for the treatment you plan to receive. Do this before making your first appointment for any kind of medical care.

The goal of this step is to make sure that you and the payer *agree in advance* about who is responsible for the costs of your medical treatment. If you think there will be more than one payer, contact all of them. Of course, there are steps you can take to resolve disagreements with a payer *after* you receive any treatment in question. However, it's far more efficient to prevent such disagreement in the first place.

If your back condition is related to a workplace injury, check with your employer immediately. This injury may involve a workers' compensation carrier, and these payers have specific rules that you must follow. For example, the carrier may limit which physicians you can see when treating the injury. In addition, you'll need to complete a First Report of Injury form. This initiates a complex series of authorizations that need to take place before you can receive covered medical care.

Finally, do not assume that a treatment will be fully covered simply because two or more payers may cover it. Those payers might

Payers for Medical Treatment Can Include

- Your health insurer
- The workers' compensation carrier for your employer
- Medicare
- Medicaid
- You
- A combination of the above

disagree and fight it out for weeks, months, or years to determine who's responsible. You could end up in the middle of this dispute. In fact, your physician or other health care provider may decline to provide the treatment you want until he or she knows that someone will pay for it.

▌ Step 4: Keep detailed records of your contacts with treatment providers and health insurers

Now is the time to start keeping complete and accurate records related to your health care and insurance. You'll depend on these records if you ever enter into a dispute with your health insurer or another payer about what's covered under your policy and how much you have to pay. Useful records will include the seven P's:

1. *People*—names and contact information (address, phone number, and e-mail address) for your health care providers, insurance agent, employee benefits manager, and other key contacts related to your health care and insurance.
2. *Policy details*—policy numbers, your current insurance card, and a complete copy of your current policy.
3. *Payments*—records of copayments, deductibles, and any other health care expenses that come out of your own pocket.
4. *Provided treatments*—dates of immunizations, lab tests, diagnostic procedures, office visits, and hospital stays.
5. *Personal correspondence*—copies of all letters, e-mail messages, claims forms, and bills relating to your health care.
6. *Phone conversations*—names, dates, and phone numbers related to calls you make to your health insurer. Document

to whom you talked, when you talked to them, and what they said. There may be times when you need to recontact people who helped you reach various financial decisions along the way. Be sure to get their names. If you don't have a name, it's as if you spoke to nobody.

7. *Personal concerns*—a log of your symptoms, medications and side effects, and questions you have for your health care provider. The idea is to get a picture of how well your treatments are working. Note any changes in your back condition and overall health over time.

Following this procedure might sound like a lot of work. It does not have to be. Just set aside a special notebook or journal for notes about your health care. Update your journal daily or weekly.

A handwritten journal can work fine, though some people like to create a computer file for this purpose. Using a computer can make it easier to edit your entries and search for specific names, dates, and other details. If you use a computer, be sure to keep backup copies of your files. Also use an envelope or folder to keep hard copies of letters, bills, and other paperwork. Whatever system you use, keep your files in a place where you can access them easily.

■ Step 5: Learn about the three stages of resolving conflict with a payer

Much of the time, people succeed in getting a health insurance plan or other payer to cover the medical treatments that they want. But sometimes disagreements arise. Your health insurer may decide that a treatment is not medically necessary or that it is simply not covered under your policy.

Often, such disputes arise over new and experimental treatments. And at other times, a treatment falls into a gray area that makes it hard to determine whether your health insurance comes into play. This can happen even with the most detailed policies. In any such case, you may quickly find yourself in conflict with a payer. Chapter 6 suggests that you adopt certain attitudes in dealing with issues related to your back care including self-empowerment, optimism, and fortitude. The same attitudes are essential to resolving conflict with a health insurer or other payer. This process can be unfriendly and time-consuming. You may need to write a series of letters or make several calls. When you call, you may be put on hold for a long time. Responses to your letters or e-mail messages may take longer than you expect.

Understandably, you may feel frustrated. Keep in mind that the time you invest to resolve disputes offers several benefits. For one, you are learning how to assert yourself in the health insurance system. And if you get a payer to agree to cover a disputed medical treatment, you could save hundred or thousands of dollars while improving your health.

At first glance, taking steps to resolve conflict with a payer might look like a hopelessly complicated task. However, resolution usually takes place in just three major stages. It's almost always wise for you to follow them in their given order.

As you seek to resolve disputes at any level, remember that you have a right to get the best health insurance you can afford and en-

Resolving Conflict with a Payer

1. An internal review conducted by your health insurer (including formal and informal appeals)
2. An external review conducted by a state agency or other independent organization
3. Legal action that you take with help from an attorney

joy complete use of its benefits. Make sure that your insurer pays the full amount it is obligated to pay for your medical care and that you avoid paying one nickel more than your policy requires.

Again, it's worthwhile to learn about these steps now even if you're not involved in a dispute with your health insurer. Be well prepared for the situation if it does arise in the future.

Note: Sometimes you can resolve a dispute relatively simply and quickly by making sure that a medical treatment was processed and billed correctly. This usually involves a telephone contact. You might only need to verify that a diagnosis code, treatment code, or related detail was supplied correctly to the insurer. Perhaps a deductible or copayment was incorrectly calculated. Correcting such clerical errors might remove the need for any kind of review or legal action.

Stage 1: Ask for an internal review

Both state and federal laws require health insurers to respond to complaints through an internal review process. It's called *internal* because the investigation is conducted by the insurer itself. The process differs across companies, but it usually includes two major steps: an informal appeal and a formal appeal.

You can begin an informal appeal simply by calling a customer service representative employed by your health insurer. As suggested earlier in this chapter, keep careful records:

- Store any paperwork related to your dispute in a file that you can find quickly.
- Whenever you talk to anyone at your health insurer's office, log the date and time of your call.
- Also write up a summary of your conversation and get the name of the person who answered your call.
- Before you hang up, ask *what* you can expect to happen next in resolving your dispute and *when* you can expect that to take

place. Note this date in your calendar and follow up if nothing happens.

If you're not satisfied with the results of an informal appeal, you can take the next step—a formal appeal. This process might also be called a *level one appeal* or *desk review*. In any case, it involves a detailed grievance process as described in your health insurance policy.

Expect at this stage to communicate more information in writing than over the phone. Also, plan to spend more time on this level of appeal. You may need to send several letters detailing the nature of your disagreement or complaint and then follow up with phone calls. The kind of information you'll need to document in writing will probably include

- Your name, address, and phone number
- Your insurance policy number, group number, or member identification number
- Your social security number
- The name, address, and phone number of any health professional who provided (or will provide) the treatment that you want to be covered by insurance
- A description of the treatment
- A statement about why the treatment is (or was) needed
- References to any sections of your policy that apply to the treatment

One key to getting the resolution you want in the least amount of time is to supply complete and accurate information at each step of a formal appeal. Any omission or inaccuracy can lead to delay. Read your policy for any time limits on making a formal appeal. Missing deadlines can result in a delay or denial of your claim.

After you've supplied the information needed for a formal appeal, you might not have further direct contact with the insurer for a while. Some insurers will review the appeal information and no-tify you in writing of their decision. Others might allow you to talk directly to the person handling your appeal.

In either case, federal laws that apply to resolving disputes with employer-sponsored health plans state that you have the right to present documents that back up your case. Federal and state laws also set time limits that the insurer must obey in responding to your appeal. In addition, your insurer must state in writing why it is denying your claim.

You might go through a formal appeal and still not get the result you want. Even so, you're still not out of options yet. The next step to take depends on your health insurer and the insurance regula-tions in your state. You might be asked to attend a hearing con-ducted before a review panel of physicians, consumers, and health plan representatives. There may be another nonbinding arbitration process for you to follow. Or your insurer may deny your claim and send a list of instructions for pursuing an external review (explained in the next section).

In any case, take full advantage of the appeals process, both in-formal and formal. Don't take the first no you receive from an in-surer as a final answer. Keep asking why a treatment was refused or a claim was denied. Then point out why you think the treatment should be covered based on the provisions of your policy.

Stage 2: Ask for an external review

Forty-one states and the District of Columbia have laws that pro-vide for external reviews (sometimes called *level two reviews*) to re-solve disputes between consumers and their health plans. This level of review involves people who are *not* representatives of your plan.

The procedure for an external review varies from state to state. In some states, you begin the process by contacting your health in-surer again. In others, you start by contacting your state insurance commissioner or another state agency. Some states contract with external review organizations (EROs) to handle this step. Your insurance commissioner or ERO will send you a list of the information you need to supply, any other actions for you to take during an external review, and the deadlines for taking those actions.

You can go online to learn more about external reviews. Check the websites for your state department of health or commissioner of insurance.

Note: You might get your health insurance from an employer or employee group that has a self-funded plan; that is, the employer or group sets aside its own money to pay for health care benefits. States are not allowed to regulate most self-funded plans, thus possibly reducing your options for an external review.

Finding out whether your health plan is self-funded can be difficult. Check your health insurance policy or ask your employee benefits manager at work. You can also contact the closest regional office of the U.S. Department of Labor. This office may also be willing to investigate any dispute that you have with a self-funded plan. If you have a disability, another possible resource is the legal protection provided under the Americans with Disabilities Act (ADA).

Stage 3: Consider legal action

It's possible that you'll exhaust the internal and external review processes without a satisfactory resolution of your dispute with a health insurer. Consider whether you have the time, energy, and money required to take further action. If your answer is yes, then your final step in most cases is to engage an attorney and take legal action.

Of course, this level of conflict resolution may require you to invest additional effort, above and beyond the work you've done for previous reviews. However, taking legal action might be worth it, especially if your claim involves a large amount of money, a treatment that could significantly improve your health, or both.

Chapter Summary:
A Checklist for Understanding Your Health Insurance

My health insurance benefits come in the form of
___ An indemnity policy
___ A managed care policy (HMO, PPO, or POS plan)
___ A self-funded plan

I have in my files the following documents relating to health insurance:
___ A summary plan description with an overview of my benefits
___ A complete copy of my policy contract
___ Copies of the insurance ID card that came with my policy
___ Contact information for my insurer's customer services department, my
employee benefits coordinator, or my insurance agent
___ Contact information for my primary care physician

I need a referral from my primary physician to
___ Consult with a spine surgeon
___ See a physical therapist
___ See another back care specialist
___ Get an MRI
___ Get a discogram
___ Get other diagnostic tests

Before making a medical appointment, I can state whether a treatment is
___ Fully covered under my policy
___ Partially covered under my policy
___ Not covered under my policy

Costs that I have to pay for health care include
___ Health insurance premiums
___ Deductibles
___ Copayments for office visits

___ Copayments for diagnostic tests
___ Copayments for surgeries and other hospital stays
___ Payments for out-of-network providers
___ Other costs

If I have duplicate coverage for a treatment, I can state
___ Which insurer will pay first
___ Which insurer will pay next
___ Which payer will be responsible for any remaining costs

I have federally mandated coverage that includes
___ Medicare Part A for hospital care
___ Medicare Part B for other medical treatments
___ Medicare Part C: Medicare+Choice
___ Medicare Part D: extended coverage for prescription drugs
___ Medicaid

I know how to resolve a dispute with my insurer including the procedures for
___ An informal appeal
___ A formal appeal
___ An external review

15

Face-to-Face with the Physical Therapist

Many back patients say they miss their old life. They miss being able to do the things they used to do. They miss moving freely and easily without discomfort or pain.

Physical therapists often play an important part in helping patients with back problems get their life back. PTs are rehabilitation experts. They focus on improving your ability to do important daily activities such as taking care of yourself, working around the house and yard, enjoying hobbies, and completing job duties. They guide you through a step-by-step treatment program to improve your mobility, increase your strength, and decrease your pain. As you move better and get stronger, you can often reclaim many of the activities you used to do. You can work toward getting your old life back.

■ What are physical therapists and what do they do?

Physical therapists are graduates of an accredited physical therapy school and have passed a national licensure examination. You might see a physical therapist at a freestanding clinic or in the physical therapy department of a hospital. Occasionally, PTs have an office in a health club.

Your physical therapy will start with an evaluation. This evaluation has three primary goals:

1. To identify where your back pain is coming from
2. To identify any conditions in your body or lifestyle that contributed to the onset of your back problem including structural abnormalities such as muscle imbalances and body movement dysfunction such as poor posture
3. To identify any musculoskeletal and movement abnormalities that have occurred as a result of your back problem such as muscle spasms and weakness

Your PT will be very interested in how you move—for example, walking, lifting, and bending—and how you function in your day-to-day life—for example, doing such things as work, household chores, personal care, and yard work.

Physical therapy is often associated with exercise. Exercise is one of the main tools PTs use to help their patients because it is the antidote to deconditioning, a common problem affecting those with back pain. Deconditioning occurs when you try to alleviate your back pain by limiting your activity level. By reducing your activities, you eventually decrease the size, strength, and flexibility of your muscles, as well as diminish your cardiovascular and muscular endurance. This often makes your condition worse.

Your physical therapist will design a reconditioning program to improve the strength and flexibility in your back and increase your overall fitness level. He or she will also help you gradually and safely reengage in your normal activities.

Physical therapy is more than just exercise. Your PT may use other skills and techniques to treat your back problem including hands-on techniques such as massage and therapeutic modalities.

PTs also spend time teaching patients how to lessen back stress by using good posture and lifting and bending correctly.

You will probably see your physical therapist more frequently early on and less frequently over time. This signifies a shift toward self-management as healing proceeds and you become more proficient and independent with your home program.

Initially, two or three physical therapy sessions each week are typical. Later, sessions will likely be scheduled once a week for a few weeks. Intermittent, infrequent visits may be scheduled long term to monitor your status and update your program.

Remember, the majority of physical therapy goes on outside the therapy clinic. Every time you sit, bend, or lift, do it right. Use the techniques you learned and practiced in physical therapy. Keep doing your home program, too.

Four to eight physical therapy sessions over a course of two to four weeks are typical for back patients. But what you learned during physical therapy can benefit your back for a lifetime.

■ Getting Referred to Physical Therapy

Typically, doctors initiate referrals to physical therapy. If they do not, you can ask for a referral. In some states, you can go to physical therapy without a doctor's referral. This is called direct access. However, the vast majority of insurance companies require a doctor's referral or they won't pay for PT services even in states with direct access.

If you don't have a doctor's referral, call the PT clinic and see if you need one. If you don't, you should still call your insurance company and ask if a doctor's referral is required to cover payment for PT services. If you can access PT directly and if your insurance doesn't require a referral, you can go ahead and schedule an appointment.

If you are referred to PT by your doctor, your therapist will work in cooperation with your physician. Your PT will communicate with your doctor as needed, sending him or her a written plan of care when you start therapy and a discharge summary of your progress when you are done.

■ Finding the Right Physical Therapist

You should put as much time and effort into finding the right PT as you would finding the right doctor. Your doctor may refer you to a specific PT clinic or a specific physical therapist. That's fine, but make sure this PT or clinic specializes in treating backs. A general PT might not be as helpful. If your doctor doesn't refer you to a PT who is a back specialist or doesn't give you a referral at all, ask for one.

If you need to find your own PT, feel free to ask friends, family, or coworkers for a recommendation. Again, however, make sure they know you need someone who specializes in backs.

You can always look in the phone book for a physical therapist. Look in the yellow pages under physical therapy. Write down the names of several clinics that are convenient for you, then call and ask if they specialize in treating back problems. If they don't, keep looking elsewhere.

You should be interested in the amount of experience your PT has with back problems. In general, PTs with more years of treating back problems have greater experience and depth of knowledge. When you schedule an appointment, ask how many years the PT has been practicing and how much of his or her practice is focused on back patients. You might get a vague answer from the office staff: "She's been around quite a while and sees a lot of back patients." That's a good enough answer. At least you know you won't be seeing someone right out of school with little experience. Ideally, you want a PT who has at least two years of experience treating backs.

When you call to schedule an appointment, you should inquire whether the same PT will see you for all your visits. Sometimes a PT will complete the initial evaluation, but a physical therapy assistant or athletic trainer will treat you after that. This is not the best situation for you. It interrupts continuity of care. It is better to see the same PT for all your appointments. If that is not possible, look for a different PT clinic.

Many therapists seek advanced certification in treating the spine. At your first appointment, you might ask your PT if she has any special certifications and how that certification was obtained. Typically, advanced certification will involve many hours of special classroom instruction as well as passing a written and hands-on examination. Advanced certification signifies that the PT is willing to go the extra mile to learn new and advanced techniques to treat the spine. Advanced certification is not a necessity when looking for a good PT, but it is a big plus.

Your physical therapist's interpersonal and communication skills are as important as her credentials and experience. You should be treated respectfully and engaged as an active partner in your physical therapy treatment plan. Your questions should be answered carefully and clearly. You should feel the PT is both caring and trustworthy.

The following list can help you determine if you are seeing the right PT. Any good physical therapist will, at a minimum, do the following:

- Ask questions and listen to your answers.
- Seek to understand your unique back problem and how it has affected your ability to be active and perform activities of daily living.
- Examine you carefully and thoroughly. You should not feel rushed through the visit.
- Describe what treatment approach he or she will use and why.
- Outline the goals of physical therapy.

- Explain what you should do if your pain flares up. You should be given an office number to call if questions arise between visits.
- Give you a written home program.
- Explain how many physical therapy sessions will likely be necessary.
- Ask if you have any questions.

■ What to Expect at Your First Visit

The physical therapist will start by asking some questions. The goal of these questions is to better understand you and your back pain.

- What are your symptoms?
- Was there a particular incident or event that brought on your symptoms?
- Are your symptoms affected by the time of day?
- What relieves your pain?
- How is your pain affected by sitting? Standing? Lying down?
- What have you tried to relieve your pain?
- What was your activity level before this injury?
- Have you had a back problem before? How did it start? What helped?
- Are you taking medications? Which ones?
- Do you have any other significant medical conditions or health concerns?

Next, your therapist will ask you to change clothes so that your back can be easily and completely examined. The examination may consist of

- Testing your sensory abilities and reflexes
- Testing your muscle strength
- Evaluating how you walk
- Checking your standing alignment
- Evaluating your range of trunk motion
- Checking the flexibility of your hip joints and important leg muscles
- Palpation (examination by touching) of the back structures and muscles

The question–answer session and the clinical examination will help identify deficits in strength, movement, flexibility, posture, structural alignment, and tissue integrity (muscle tightness, ligament tenderness, etc.). After the examination, your PT will design a treatment program. Most often, treatment begins on the first visit. Sometimes, however, the PT will take time to review the findings and start treatment on the next visit.

The PT will sit down with you and discuss your treatment program—what it entails and why. She will tell you what results to expect and how long treatment should take. If there is anything you don't understand, ask.

Stay focused and attentive in any discussion you have with your physical therapist. Careful listening will help you better understand what will occur in physical therapy and why. You can also request a written summary of important findings and the plan of care. Or request the names of books or other written resources that will help you better understand your condition, the treatment plan, and the expected recovery.

∎ Physical Therapy Treatment

In designing your treatment program, the PT will draw on an understanding of the science of tissue healing, the adaptive changes the body undergoes as a result of pain and immobility, the influence of exercise and reconditioning on the healing process, and the important anatomy of the back and related areas. The cornerstones of physical therapy treatment for back pain are education, exercise, hands-on techniques, and modalities.

Education

Most of us take sitting, standing, and bending for granted. Not so when your back is painful. Doing these activities wrong can make back pain worse and possibly even hinder recovery. In physical therapy you learn to do these activities in a way that causes the least stress to the painful area.

• Proper posture can help eliminate back pain and prevent its reoccurrence. Good standing posture is comfortable and balanced, supporting upright alignment without stress and strain. Sitting posture is also important, especially since more than half of today's workforce has a job where they sit for most of the day. Good alignment, a good chair, and appropriate support can minimize stress on your back. Your PT might recommend a back support such as a lumbar roll (a small cushion that supports your back while sitting).

• Lifting and bending are two movements often associated with the onset of back pain. Your PT will teach you how to do these movements correctly, reducing stress to your back.

• Ergonomics is the study of how your body interacts with its environment at work, during sports, and in other settings. Your PT will review the ergonomics of your day—your work habits, workstation setup, and recreational/sports routine. The goal is to eliminate unhealthy postures or movements so that your back can get healthy again and stay that way.

Exercise

Exercise is the heart and soul of physical therapy. The specific exercises prescribed for you depend on several factors including your diagnosis, stage of healing, age, fitness level, and identified deficits.

• Which exercises are best for the patient with acute lower back pain and some leg pain? This is a common situation for which a physical therapist is requested. There are various schools of therapy such as the McKenzie school and the Williams school, but a good therapist will carefully evaluate which positions and movements are painful and which are not. He or she can then design an exercise program that focuses on the nonpainful movements. A rigid focus on one school or another is not the way to go.

• Strengthening exercises are used to address weak muscles. Muscle weakness may have been present before your back problem began and may have contributed to its onset. Or weakness may be a consequence of your back problem, resulting from a limited activity level. (This is called secondary weakness.) Reconditioning important muscles, including the abdominals, back stabilizers, and gluteal muscles, is critical for a healthy spine. Strong muscles can minimize harmful stresses to the spine, prepare the back for increased activity, and help prevent reinjury.

• Stretching exercises are used when tight or inflexible muscles are present. Tight muscles create awkward stresses on the spine. Regaining muscle flexibility helps restore health to the back. The hip flexors and hamstrings are two muscles that often need stretching when the back is painful.

Not only will your PT teach you what exercises to do—he or she will also teach you how to exercise correctly. Pacing involves a gradual increase in activity according to a predetermined plan. Pacing helps keep you from overdoing it and suffering a setback or flare-up. In addition, your PT will instruct you to

- Go slowly, emphasizing quality over quantity.
- Pay attention to your body so that you can feel what you are doing.
- Breathe slowly, smoothly, and easily. Never hold your breath while exercising.

Hands-On Techniques

Physical therapists employ many different hands-on techniques that can benefit the back patient.

- Soft tissue mobilization involves vigorous massaging to release spasms, increase circulation, and improve extensibility (the ability of a tissue to move easily).
- Joint mobilizations may be used when restricted segmental motion (motion between two adjacent vertebrae) or other joint motion restrictions are noted.
- Muscle energy techniques (METs) are used to restore normal position and motion to the lumbar segments and sacroiliac joints. With METs, the physical therapist applies resistance to contraction of specific muscles while the patient is prepositioned to facilitate correct movement of segments or joints.

Modalities

Therapeutic modalities are sometimes used in physical therapy to effect tissue healing.

- Hot packs are used to increase circulation to an area.
- Cold packs are used to diminish pain, especially after exercising.

- Mechanical traction uses a mechanical device to create traction, or separation, of the vertebrae in the spine. Though popular a decade or so ago, mechanical traction is used infrequently now.

Home Program

Your therapist will probably give you a list of instructions and exercises or positioning movements to do at home. This home program is an extension of your physical therapy sessions and should be carried out diligently. This will help ensure the best possible results.

Let's face it—exercising can be monotonous. It requires discipline to stick with an exercise program, but the payoff is a healthier back.

Written instructions and diagrams of exercises work best for home programs. Once you walk out the door, it is hard to remember exactly what you are supposed to do. If your physical therapist doesn't give you written instructions and exercise handouts, ask for them.

▍ Evidence-Based Physical Therapy

PTs use many techniques to treat back problems, but some of these approaches have better evidence to support their efficacy than others. One of the best ways a physical therapist can help you recover from back pain is by teaching you appropriate exercises. Therapeutic exercise, including stretching, strengthening, and mobility exercises, has solid evidence to support its benefit in alleviating back pain and improving function, especially in those with subacute (lasting four to twelve weeks) and chronic back pain (lasting more than twelve weeks).

In addition, there is good evidence to support the use of muscle energy techniques, mobilization, and back education (learning proper posture, lifting, bending). The jury is still out on the effectiveness of mechanical traction, thermotherapy (such as hot packs), massage/myofascial release, and electrical muscle stimulation. Therapeutic ultrasound, biofeedback, and transcutaneous electrical nerve stimulation (TENS) generally show no clinical benefit.

In summary, the most effective physical therapy approaches are

- Stretching exercises
- Strengthening exercises
- Mobility exercises
- Aerobic exercises
- Muscle energy techniques
- Mobilization
- Back care education (posture, lifting, bending)

Approaches that may be helpful are

- Thermotherapy
- Mechanical traction
- Massage/myofascial release

Approaches with no supportive evidence are

- Therapeutic ultrasound
- Transcutaneous electrical nerve stimulation (TENS)
- Biofeedback

Most physical therapy patients will benefit from a focus on those approaches with the strongest supportive evidence. Your physical therapist will probably use these treatment approaches in combination with others for the best results.

▌ Diagnosis-Specific Physical Therapy

Your diagnosis distinctly affects your physical therapy treatment. It tells the PT what is wrong with your back, which in turn dictates the kind of treatment that will work best. For example, back extension exercises are often effective in treating a disc herniation, but extension exercises are not recommended for spinal stenosis.

Our information gives you a general idea of what to expect in PT based on your diagnosis. It describes the way PTs commonly treat back problems. Your PT will follow these guidelines in tailoring your treatment program to your particular needs.

Spinal Stenosis

Patients with spinal stenosis have limited trunk extension—they cannot bend backward at the trunk because it increases the nerve pinching, and they often cannot stand upright. PT typically consists of

- Lumbar flexion exercises such as knee to chest
- Strengthening of the abdominal muscles
- Strengthening of any leg muscles that have become weak
- Stretching of the hip flexors
- General conditioning via stationary cycling
- Patient education that covers such topics as avoiding prolonged walking and standing and carrying heavy loads

Muscle Sprain/Strain

The first PT goal is alleviating muscle tension and soreness. Next, the patient begins strengthening and reconditioning. Treatment includes

- Modalities such as heat or cold packs to the sore, tight muscles

- Strengthening to the core muscles: back, abdominal, and gluteal
- Stretching to tight leg muscles, especially the hamstrings and hip flexors
- Education regarding good posture, proper body mechanics, and general spine health

Spondylolisthesis

Physical therapy for spondylolisthesis focuses on training the muscles in the spine to better stabilize and control the spine. Treatment may consist of

- Postural training to maintain a neutral spine position, avoiding the extremes of flexion and extension
- Strengthening exercises for the back and abdominal muscles
- Functional training to perform daily activities with a neutral spine position
- Patient education focused on avoiding a prolonged flexed posture, maintaining good posture, using a lumbar support, and using a supportive chair

Disc Herniation

Disc herniation typically causes lower back pain with pain and/or tingling in the back of the thigh to the lower leg or possibly the foot. PT focuses on treating these symptoms via

- McKenzie or Williams exercises
- Posture and body mechanics training that avoids trunk flexion and prolonged sitting
- Ergonomic training that teaches how to lift without flexing the trunk
- Strengthening and general conditioning as needed

- Massage and modalities to relieve muscle spasms caused by pain
- Unloading the spine by using swimming pool exercises

Disc Degeneration

Disc degeneration can cause a loss of structural stability in the spine. PT focuses on training the muscles to better work as spine stabilizers—for example,

- Postural training to maintain a neutral spine and avoid extreme flexion or extension
- Strengthening to the back muscles that contribute to spine stabilization
- Stretching to the hip flexors and hamstrings
- Abdominal and gluteal muscle strengthening
- Training in maintaining a neutral spine position during functional activities such as sitting, bending, and lifting

Osteoporosis

This condition is characterized by a risk for bone fractures, and the spine is one area where these fractures often occur. PT typically includes

- Posture training for improved spine alignment
- Strengthening exercises to increase back muscle strength (stronger back muscles are associated with a lower risk for back fracture)
- Safe strengthening of the abdominal muscles that avoids trunk flexion
- Instructions in avoiding a rounded spine during daily activities and in avoiding jarring the spine
- Instructions in minimizing the risk of falling

Scoliosis

There is no scientific evidence that PT has any value for scoliosis treatment.

Scheuermann's Disease

There is no scientific evidence that PT has any value for the treatment of Scheuermann's disease.

Pre- and Postsurgical PT

Presurgical PT focuses on strengthening exercises, body mechanics, and educational topics that will help prepare you for a successful surgical outcome. Postsurgical PT includes proper care for your back after surgery and guidance in increasing your activity level. PT will probably include

- Instruction in posture, body mechanics, and ergonomics
- Graded strengthening exercises for the back and legs
- Appropriate stretching exercises
- Instruction in how to do normal activities such as bending, lifting, getting in and out of bed, sitting in a chair, and riding in a car
- General fitness, typically a walking program

▮ No pain, no gain? No way!

Physical therapy should not increase your back pain. However, because therapists work hard to balance the need for activity with the need for healing, occasionally a brief flare-up might occur. If it does, apply a cold pack or ice to the painful area for ten to fifteen minutes every hour or two until the pain subsides. Exercise is often put on hold during a flare-up. Make your therapist aware of flare-ups and ask whether your treatment plan should be amended.

Exercises may cause soreness in the muscles that are being worked. This is a normal consequence of reconditioning weak muscles. This soreness is transitory, vague, and located in the muscles (not the tendons or joints). It will go away in a few days, leaving behind stronger, better conditioned muscles. Again, tell your therapist about this muscle soreness and follow his or her guidance.

You and your physical therapist can work as a powerful team in helping your back problem. However, if physical therapy is not bringing the expected results, return to your family practice doctor or the physician who referred you.

16

Face-to-Face with the Medical Specialists

One of the best things you can do before your appointment with a specialist is review Chapter 6. Seeing a highly educated and specially trained doctor can be intimidating. When medical terms are part of the conversation, it is easy to get confused. It's hard to keep everything straight when there are a lot of questions to answer.

So before you see the specialist,

- Learn as much as you can about the spine. If you have a diagnosis, learn more about your condition.
- Write down questions you have for the doctor.
- Approach your appointment with an optimistic mindset. Bring a feeling of empowerment, too. Be determined to bring about the best outcome for yourself.

When you're at the appointment,

- Listen attentively.
- Ask questions if you don't understand something.
- Request written materials if you need more information.

▌ Getting Recommendations to the Medical Specialist

In most cases, your primary care doctor will manage your case, referring you to the appropriate back care specialists as you need them. When you get referrals to specialists or surgeons, ask for a few names so that you can compare credentials and experience. Referrals are not always based on merit. Friendship and social connections sometimes play a factor. Don't assume the doctor knows all the best people. Use the information presented later in this chapter to check out any doctor you might see.

If you need to find a specialist on your own, networking—tapping into the knowledge and experience of people you know—can help you find a good doctor. Ask friends, family, and coworkers for recommendations. You probably won't have to look far to find a person you know who has or has had back pain. Someone who has been down the same road you are on might have a good recommendation. Trying these two simple steps can help you find the right person with the right recommendation:

1. Find someone whose back pain problems have come to a happy ending. This may seem obvious, but the people who know the best professionals are usually those who got better. Don't talk to your brother-in-law who has seen a dozen different specialists and is still miserable. Talk to someone whose back pain was resolved with the skilled help of his or her doctor.

2. Compare apples with apples. The back is complex, and pain can arise from many different parts of the spine. Someone whose back problem is most like yours is the best place to start looking for a recommendation. Talk to someone about your age whose back problem came on in a similar manner and whose symptoms are comparable. If you are 25 years old and recently hurt your back playing football, your 80-year-old grandmother with years of chronic back pain is not a good source for a recommendation. But a coworker who injured his back playing soccer might be.

Friends or family who work in the medical profession are another source to tap for recommendations. If your sister is an operating room nurse, call her. If your neighbor is a hospital administrator, call him.

• If you have recently moved to a new area, ask your former doctor for a referral. Or if you see a different kind of doctor regularly, such as a gynecologist or your child's pediatrician, you might seek a referral there.

• Hospitals often offer a referral service with the names of staff doctors. The referral service cannot, however, vouch for the quality of the physician's care. Also, the hospital will not recommend a doctor who does not work at its facility, no matter how good the doctor may be. Ask for the names of several doctors, then compare credentials and experience.

• Most health care plans have a directory of physicians listed by specialty. Finding doctors from that directory means they are covered by your insurance plan, which, unfortunately, has nothing to do with how good they are. Again, do your homework and check out the credentials and experience of the doctors on the list.

▌ Networking to Get an Appointment

Once you find the right doctor, getting an appointment may be your next hurdle. The best doctors are in high demand, and getting an appointment can take time. Start by calling the general scheduling line. If the first available appointment is too far away, try networking. If you know someone who might have a relative or friend in the physician's office, see if that person might put in a word for you.

Talk to as many people as you can. You don't know who might surprise you with a connection and an offer to help. One gentleman found the connection he needed by talking to a neighbor in the elevator of his apartment building.

If a physician referred you to the doctor, try calling back and seeing if he or she might help. A phone call from a doctor might get you past all kinds of scheduling red tape.

Without connections, stay persistent and flexible. Remind yourself to keep the right mindset—staying optimistic and displaying forbearance while holding to the belief that you will find a solution. Ask if you might leave your cell phone number for any last-minute cancellations. You might also ask if the doctor has partners with similar treatment philosophies and success rates or if the doctor has trained any other nearby specialists. If you are comfortable seeing one of those doctors, you might be able to get an appointment sooner.

▌ Face-to-Face with the Rehabilitation Physician

Rehabilitation physicians practice a medical specialty called physical medicine and rehabilitation (PM&R). The physicians who specialize in PM&R are called physiatrists.

The physiatrist will work to improve your function by treating you directly, leading a team of different health care professionals or acting as a consultant. Physiatrists practice nonsurgical medicine and distinguish themselves from other medical practitioners by focusing on the whole person, addressing physical, emotional, psychosocial, and vocational needs.

Physiatrists practice in rehabilitation settings, hospitals, and private offices. They often have broad practices, but they may specialize in one area such as back problems.

Checking Out the Physiatrist

Even if you are referred to a physiatrist by another doctor, it is worth checking out some basic information before your first appointment.

• Make certain the physiatrist regularly treats patients with back problems. You don't want to see a physiatrist who specializes in stroke rehabilitation. Simply ask whether the doctor regularly treats back problems when you schedule your first appointment. Most general physiatrists do.

• Check to see if the physiatrist is covered by your insurance plan. You can look in your health plan directory or call your insurance plan. You can also ask the doctor's office if your type of insurance is accepted.

If you need to find a physiatrist without the help of a referral from your doctor, you might start by asking family, friends, and coworkers. Be sure they understand you need a doctor who treats back problems.

You can also use your local telephone directory. Look under the heading "physicians." They are often listed by specialty, so look under "physical medicine and rehabilitation." Again, when you call to make an appointment, ask whether the doctor regularly treats back problems.

Finally, you can receive a printed list of board-certified physiatrists in your area by calling 312-464-9700 or by sending an e-mail to awatson@aapmr.org.

What to Expect at the First Visit

The physiatrist will take a history including questions about your back problem and your health in general. The doctor will also be interested in how your back problem has affected your job, your sense of well-being, and your social life.

Next, the doctor will perform a detailed clinical examination. You will be asked to change clothes so that your spine and legs can be seen. The examination will be very similar to the one performed by your primary care doctor though more comprehensive.

If necessary, the physiatrist may order or perform further diagnostic tests. Physiatrists use the same diagnostic tools as other physicians (X-rays, CAT scan, MRI, etc.), but they also use several special techniques referred to as electrodiagnostic testing. This testing helps the doctor diagnose conditions that cause pain, weakness, and numbness.

Electrodiagnostic tests include electromyography (EMG), nerve conduction studies, and somatosensory evoked potential (SSEP).

• An **EMG** is recommended to assess the function of a nerve. If a nerve is pinched, electrical conduction along it slows. This test involves placing small needles in the muscles, which can be uncomfortable but poses no major health risks.

• **Nerve conduction studies** test the response of the nerves in the legs or arms to electrical stimulation. The results help determine if a nerve is damaged or compromised.

• **SSEPs** assess the speed of electrical conduction across the spinal cord. If the spinal cord is pinched, the electrical signals will travel slower than usual. Since the spinal cord ends before the lumbar spine, this test is not used for lumbar spine problems.

The physiatrist will synthesize the information from your history, physical examination, and diagnostic tests to arrive at a diagnosis (or to confirm the one given to you by your primary care doctor) and determine a plan of care. The doctor will discuss both the diagnosis and treatment plan with you (occasionally this is done with a telephone call). Listen carefully. If something is unclear, ask for more information. You may also inquire if written materials are available that explain your diagnosis and the recommended treatment.

How Physiatrists Treat Back Problems

The treatment plan prescribed by your physiatrist may include

- Medications
- Active physical therapy such as self-management skills, exercise, body mechanics, and postural exercises
- Passive therapeutic modalities such as heat, cold, electrical stimulation, and so on
- A back brace
- Cortisone injections of ligaments, muscles, bursae, or joints
- Referrals to other nonphysician health care professionals such as a physical therapists, occupational therapists, or psychology and vocational rehabilitation specialists
- A referral to a spine surgeon

Physiatrists may treat patients in their office. Most often, physiatrists refer patients with back pain to other health care professionals including

- Physical therapists for restoring movement and strength through education, exercises, and hands-on techniques
- Occupational therapists to improve ability to perform daily activities safely and efficiently and to recommend home and job adaptations
- Vocational rehabilitation specialists to help with the transition back to work or to assist patients in finding new jobs that suit their physical limitations
- Psychologists to help assess and treat psychosocial needs.

The physiatrist then serves as the leader of this treatment team, communicating and collaborating with each team member to ensure integrated care. The physiatrist will continue to see you intermittently to monitor your recovery.

Do you have the right physiatrist?

A good physiatrist will exhibit the attributes of a good doctor as listed in Chapter 10. In addition, a good physiatrist should be interested in you as a whole person. He or she should explore how your back pain is affecting you socially and emotionally and how your job performance has been impacted.

You should expect the physiatrist to take a detailed history and to perform a thorough examination. He or she should be interested in finding the source of your back pain and treating it aggressively.

Most of all, you should trust your physiatrist. You should feel confident that he or she cares about your back problem and will work with you to find the best way to treat it. The doctor should treat you respectfully, listening carefully to your questions and spending adequate time with you.

■ Face-to-Face with the Spine Specialist

Spine specialists are medical doctors (MD or DO) who devote their practice to the care of patients with spine problems. They come from several different medical specialties including physiatry (physical medicine and rehabilitation), orthopedic surgery, neurology, and neurosurgery. Some spine specialists such as physiatrists practice nonsurgical medicine. Others practice both nonsurgical and surgical spine care, functioning both as spine specialists and spine surgeons.

Spine specialists spend 90% to 100% of their time with back patients. They are interested in the latest literature and research about the spine. They attend professional meetings to keep up with new developments. They know the latest in diagnosing and treating the spine. They are the spine experts.

A visit with a spine specialist is indicated if you are still hurting after seeing your primary care doctor and maybe receiving physical therapy. You may need to see a spine specialist if you have moved out of the acute back problem phase and are now in the subacute or chronic phase.

Checking Out the Spine Specialist

Before you schedule an appointment with a spine specialist, here are several important considerations:

• Double-check whether the doctor's practice focuses on spine patients. Just ask if the doctor sees mostly back patients when you schedule your first appointment.

• Ask about the doctor's experience. Ask the scheduler or perhaps the doctor's nurse how many years the doctor has been practicing as a spine specialist.

• Check to see if your insurance plan covers visits with this doctor. You can look in your health plan directory or call your insurance company.

• Ask about the doctor's hospital affiliation. Your appointment with the spine specialist will take place in his office, but you might be referred to the hospital for a procedure or test. You might want to make sure the hospital is one you are comfortable with and one that is reasonably convenient.

What to Expect at the First Visit

The spine specialist will probably ask you to fill out a basic questionnaire. Then he will complete a detailed history, perform a physical examination, and review any X-rays or lab tests you've already had done. If indicated, the doctor may order further X-rays or tests. His main initial objective will be to determine a specific diagnosis or confirm the diagnosis you've already been given. Along with your physical problem, the spine specialist will be interested in your mental and social situation. These factors influence your pain.

At the conclusion of your first visit (or maybe at your second visit if lab results are pending), your doctor will arrive at a diagnosis and will share that information with you. Make sure you

- Completely understand your diagnosis. If it has a confusing name that is hard to remember, ask the doctor to write it down.
- Know what your diagnosis means.
- Ask what the natural course of your condition is if it is left un-treated.

How Spine Specialists Treat Back Problems

Once he arrives at a diagnosis, the doctor will devise a logical treatment plan. You might have a problem that is clearly nonsurgi-cal or one for which a period of nonsurgical care should be at-tempted first. The spine specialist will provide the right nonsurgical care.

Good spine specialists will use many different treatment ap-proaches. In addition, they will access the expertise of other doctors and health care providers. For example, if you are diagnosed with spinal stenosis, you might be referred to a radiologist for a series of epidural steroid injections (injections of medicine directly into the spine). If disc degeneration is the source of your back problem, you might be referred to physical therapy for a special therapy program. If you have severe chronic pain but are not a surgical candidate, you might be referred to a chronic pain specialist.

Once your doctor has proposed a treatment plan, make sure you understand

- Your treatment options
- The risks and benefits of each treatment option
- Why the doctor is recommending a specific type of treatment

Do you have the right spine specialist?

In addition to following the guidelines of a good physician as listed on pages 112–113, a good spine specialist will

- Be committed to arriving at a specific diagnosis for your back problem
- Thoroughly explain your treatment options and offer a strong rationale for recommending a certain treatment
- Avoid the overuse of narcotic medications
- Recognize when surgery might be appropriate and refer you to a spine surgeon (if your doctor is a nonsurgical spine specialist)

If you are dissatisfied with how the spine specialist manages your back problem, don't just give up. Try another doctor. Ask your primary care doctor if she can refer you to a different spine specialist. Above all, don't settle for an endless course of narcotic medications. That is not the solution to your back problem.

▌ Face-to-Face with the Spine Surgeon

Like spine specialists, spine surgeons devote 90% or more of their practice to the care of patients with back problems. They are distinguished in being trained to perform spine surgery. Spine surgeons are either orthopedic spine surgeons or neurosurgical spine surgeons. Along with medical school and four to five years of residency, these doctors have completed a spine fellowship—an additional year focused solely on spine training. A typical spine surgeon has ten years of training after completing college.

Finding the Right Spine Surgeon

Spine surgeons are not equally competent in every different surgical procedure for the spine. Just as there are many things that can go wrong with the spine, there are many different surgical procedures to correct these problems. For example, when surgery is indicated for patients with spinal stenosis, they undergo a procedure called decompression (see page 57). A diagnosis of spondylolisthesis might be addressed with a surgical procedure called spinal fusion (see pages 60–66). Spine surgeons focus on certain surgical procedures based on training.

Traditionally, neurosurgical spine surgeons have focused on spinal decompression and have done few spine fusion procedures. By contrast, orthopedic spine surgeons have focused on spine fusion procedures and only some of the decompression procedures. Recently, some of these training differences have faded, but most spine surgeons continue to specialize in certain procedures.

You need to be sure your spine surgeon specializes in and has experience with the specific surgical procedure you need. If your surgeon recommends surgery for you, ask him how much experience he has with the recommended procedure.

Trusting someone to operate on your spine is no small matter. Be sure your surgeon makes you feel comfortable and establishes good rapport. In addition, he should

- Encourage questions
- Educate you about the recommended surgery
- Encourage a second opinion
- Make sure that good conservative treatment has been carried out appropriately and for an adequate amount of time before surgery is recommended

Does a referral to a spine surgeon mean I need surgery?

Spine surgeons perform surgery on only a small minority of the patients they see. For example, the Twin Cities Spine Center (consisting of only fellowship-trained orthopedic spine surgeons) sees about fifteen thousand patients per year. Only two thousand of these patients (about 13%) end up having surgery.

Surgeons are always in the best position to determine whether the patient needs surgery. They know firsthand the results of such procedures. The spine surgeon will perform a detailed examination to determine the appropriate treatment for you. He might refer you back to your original doctor (the one who referred you to the spine surgeon). He might treat you nonoperatively. Or he might schedule you for surgery either immediately or in the future.

What to Expect at the First Visit

You should expect a thorough evaluation including a questionnaire for your completion, your history taken by the surgeon, a physical examination, and a review of any imaging studies (X-rays, MRI, CAT scan) you brought with you or had sent ahead. If you need further imaging studies or lab tests, the surgeon will order them.

At the end of your first visit or after the results of additional studies or tests have been reviewed, the surgeon will discuss your diagnosis and treatment options with you. Then he will recommend a specific treatment for your back problem.

If a nonsurgical treatment is recommended, be sure you understand

- Your treatment options
- The risks and benefits of each treatment option
- Why the doctor is recommending a specific type of treatment

If surgery is recommended, learn as much as you can from the surgeon about the procedure including

- Exactly what is done in the operation
- The possible risks and the likelihood of them happening (Are they $\frac{1}{1000}$, $\frac{1}{100}$, $\frac{1}{10}$?)
- The typical outcome
- How you get ready for surgery
- The typical course after surgery
- Alternative options if you choose not to have surgery

If you think it would be helpful, ask the surgeon for the name and phone number of one of his patients who has had the same surgery that you might have. Hearing a firsthand report of another's experience can help you better understand what to expect.

Do I have to have surgery if it is recommended?

You do not have to follow a surgeon's recommendation to have surgery. Spine surgery is almost always elective—meaning you and the surgeon elect when to do the surgery. If you choose not to have recommended surgery, be absolutely sure you understand the consequences of that decision.

Sometimes back surgery is truly an emergency. Dr. Winter had a case in which a woman was brought by ambulance from an outlying hospital. She had an infection in the spine that was pressing on the spinal cord and causing paralysis. She was taken immediately (in the middle of the night) to the operating room for surgery. A delay of even a few hours would have resulted in permanent paralysis for this woman. However, this situation is an exception. Most spine surgeries are not emergencies.

In almost all cases, you should get a second opinion regarding a proposed spine surgery. Don't be afraid this will hurt the doctor's feelings—all good surgeons are happy to have you seek a second opinion. Sometimes the second surgeon will agree with the first surgeon. Other times, she might recommend a different type of treatment or a different kind of surgery. In this case, you will need further discussions with both surgeons to find the reason for their differences. Or you might even get a third opinion.

Getting a Second Opinion

Your primary care doctor might be the best source for the name of a spine surgeon for a second opinion. You can call the office and ask for a recommendation. You can also ask family, friends, and coworkers for recommendations. Just be sure they understand you need a spine surgeon.

Don't seek a second opinion from a doctor in the same medical group as the first spine surgeon. You are more likely to get a fresh perspective from a doctor who is not affiliated with the first surgeon.

17

Taking Control When You Need Surgery

A lot needs to happen between the time you decide to have surgery and the actual surgery date. You can increase your chances for successful surgery by careful and thorough preparation. Throughout your preparations, keep a take-charge mindset. If you have questions, ask them. If you need more information, ask the surgeon, the nurse, or the physician's assistant. What is described below is a scenario for a fairly major spine procedure such as a multi-level decompression or a fusion. Shorter and less complex surgeries can be quite different. For example, a simple laminotomy and disc fragment removal is most often done as an outpatient procedure or at the most, an overnight stay. Preparing for successful surgery involves five steps:

1. Getting your mind and body ready
2. Readying your home
3. Setting up a support system
4. Preparing for your hospital stay
5. Learning the most in the hospital

■ Step 1: Getting Your Mind and Body Ready for Surgery

Being Comfortable with Your Decision to Have Surgery

Back surgery is almost always elective. Even though a surgeon recommends it, you have a choice whether to have the surgery. Deciding to have back surgery is a serious consideration. The following questions will help you decide whether surgery is right for you at this time. Or if you have already decided to have surgery, thinking about these issues can affirm your decision.

1. Have you given adequate time and effort to nonsurgical treatment options? If you have worked your way up the Back Care Pyramid and carefully followed the advice of your primary care doctor, physical therapist, and spine specialist but continue to have significant pain, surgery may be your best option.

2. Are your symptoms interfering with your life? If your back problem is making it harder for you to move and function, do your job, and participate in the activities you enjoy, surgery may be right for you at this time.

3. Have you met with a recommended and credentialed spine surgeon and received satisfactory information about

- *What surgery is planned and what it entails?*
- *What the surgeon's success rate is with this specific surgery?*
- *What the possible complications are and the likelihood that they might happen?*
- *How long the surgery will take and how long you will be in the hospital?*
- *How long it will be until you feel really good?*
- *How long you will be out of work or school, how long*

until you can drive, and how long until you can do house and yard work?

- *The type of aftercare you might need (extra help in the home or a transitional care unit/rehabilitation center)?*
- *Alternative options if you do not have the recommended surgery?*

Satisfactory information about these topics is critical in helping you make an informed decision about surgery.

4. Do you have a realistic grasp of your surgery outcome? Surgery will alter your spine, ultimately leading to a "new normal." In all likelihood, your pain will improve but not totally disappear.

5. Have you gotten a second or even third opinion about surgery? Getting a second (or even third) opinion can help clarify the exact nature of your back problem and your best treatment options including whether surgery is right for you.

Setting a Surgery Date

Carefully consider your work and social obligations when you set a surgery date. You will need several weeks off work to recover from *major* spine surgery. Other surgeries require less time off. Pick a time when it is easiest to be away from your job.

You will also need the help of family and friends for shopping and household tasks during recovery. Setting up a schedule of who can help and when can set your mind at ease and assure you that you will be cared for.

Getting a Presurgical Physical Examination

You will need to meet with your primary care doctor for a presurgical examination. He will make sure your heart and lungs are healthy enough for your specific surgery. He will also review the medications you are taking as well as any vitamins or herbal substances. Certain types of medications must be stopped before surgery (such as aspirin, antiinflammatory medications, and blood thinners). Your doctor will tell you which medications to stop and when. Write this information down so that you won't forget.

If you are having significant pain and are concerned about how to manage it until surgery, talk to your primary care doctor or spine surgeon at this time. He or she might recommend an over-the-counter medication or write a prescription.

If you are a smoker, the doctor can give you advice on how to quit before surgery. Be aware that some spine surgeons will not do elective fusion surgery until you have been completely off nicotine for at least three months.

Your primary care doctor will mail or fax the results of your presurgical examination to your surgeon. It might be helpful to request a copy of the report as well as copies of any tests your surgeon requested before surgery. You can bring those copies with you to the hospital on the day of surgery just to make sure they get there.

Mental Preparation

Mental preparation for surgery begins with accurate information and realistic expectations. Get as much information as you need to remove anxiety about the "unknowns." Also, be realistic about the seriousness of spine surgery. Spine operations can be complex. Do not expect to wake up from surgery feeling energized. It will take time—typically a couple of days—to recover from the anesthesia and the stress your body underwent during surgery. Fortunately, your health care team will be there to help every step of the way.

Remind yourself how the right mindset can make surgery and recovery successful. Continue to use empowerment, believing nothing will happen before or after surgery that you don't have the ability and resources to deal with. As a hospital patient, you are legally entitled to certain rights. You have the right to accurate information, the right to privacy, the right to be your own decision maker, and the right to refuse or consent to treatment. Don't be a passive patient. Be involved in your care. Actively participate in all important decisions.

In addition to empowerment, stay optimistic, believing you have made the right decision and that you will have a successful result. Have fortitude, too. When things don't go absolutely smoothly—and they probably won't—be willing to accept the ups and downs.

Relaxation exercises can help if you become anxious or feel tense. Mental or emotional stress can often cause muscle tension, which in turn can lead to pain. Take a few minutes and breathe deeply and slowly, inhaling through your nose and exhaling through your mouth. Or pause briefly to close your eyes and imagine a relaxing scene—a quiet lake or a peaceful sunset. Chapter 18 has more detailed relaxation exercises.

Physical Preparation

Your surgeon or physical therapist may have given you some exercises to do before surgery. It is important to be as active as possible before surgery, so carefully follow the program recommended to you. If you were not given a presurgical exercise program, ask your surgeon if it is okay to use the one outlined below.

Try to do each to these exercises 5 times. If an exercise is easy, add 5 repetitions each week until you reach 20 (5 repetitions of each exercise the first week, 10 repetitions the second week, 15 the third week, 20 the fourth week; continue with 20 repetitions until surgery). Do the exercise program twice daily. If one of the exercises causes back pain, stop doing it.

Ankle Pumps Bend your ankles up, bringing your toes toward your knees. Then bend both ankles down, pointing your toes. Up and down once is 1 repetition.

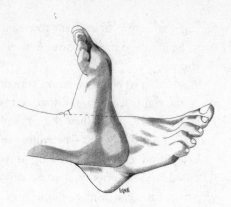

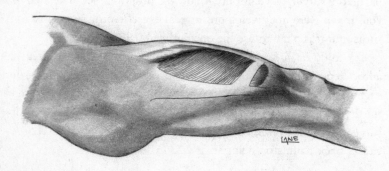

Thigh Squeeze On your bed (or floor) as comfortable for you, lie flat on your back and tighten the muscles along the top of both of your thighs by pushing the back of your knee into the bed. Hold 5 seconds, then relax.

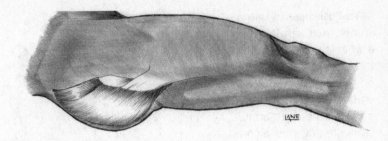

Buttock Squeeze Lying flat on your back on your bed (or floor), tighten your buttock muscles by squeezing the muscles together. Hold 5 seconds and release.

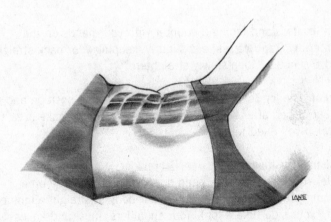

Abdominal Sets Lie on your back on your bed or floor with both knees bent. Tighten your stomach muscles, pulling your belly button toward your spine. Don't move the spine—avoid arching it up or flattening it down. Hold 5 seconds, then release.

Chair Push-Ups Sit in a sturdy chair with arms or a wheelchair with the brakes locked. Set your feet flat on the floor and your hands on the chair arms. Push down on the chair arms, straightening your elbows so that your buttocks lift off the chair seat. (If you need to, use your legs to help.) Hold 5 seconds, then release.

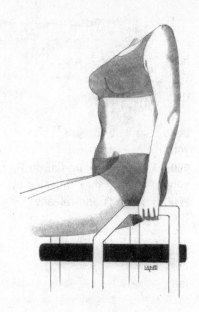

Mini-Squats Stand facing a counter with your hands on the countertop. Bend your knees slightly, keeping your back straight. Hold 5 seconds, then slowly straighten.

Log Roll The log roll is the correct way to change position and to get out of bed after surgery. Practicing it now will make it easy to do when you need to.

To change positions:
While lying on your back, bend one knee up, then the other. Keeping your knees together and your body in straight alignment, roll to your side (like a log). Your shoulders, hips, and knees should all move together.

To get out of bed:
Roll to your side as described above. Slide your body to the edge of the bed. Lower your feet to the floor as you push away from the bed.

Breathing Exercises

Breathing exercises are simple but extremely important. They help prevent postsurgery breathing problems and complications such as pneumonia. Practice these exercises now so that you can do them well after surgery.

Deep Breathing Breathe in deeply through your nose—your chest and abdomen should expand as you breathe in. Hold your breath for 5 to 10 counts. Slowly let your breath out through your mouth. Rest, then repeat 10 times.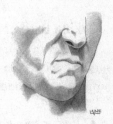

Coughing Breathe in deeply through your nose. Breathe out through your mouth, letting your chest sink down and in as you do. Take a second breath in the same way. Take a third breath. This time, hold your breath momentarily, then cough as hard as you can, forcing all the air out of your lungs. Repeat 2 more times.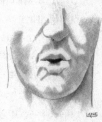

All exercises in this chapter are excerpted/adapted from Understanding Your Spine Surgery, *2nd ed. Copyright 2002, Allina Health System, with permission from Allina Health System Press.*

Healthy Eating

Eating a healthy diet can help prepare your body for the challenge of back surgery and the rigors of recovery. A healthy diet should emphasize

- A variety of fiber-rich fruits and vegetables each day
- Whole grains
- Protein from lean meat, fish, and eggs

- Less than 10% of calories from saturated fats
- Limiting total fat to 25% to 30% of calories and emphasizing polyunsaturated fats from nuts, fish, and vegetable oils
- Three servings per day of low-fat dairy products
- Drinking liberal amounts of water and noncaffeinated beverages

Taking Care of Presurgical Business

Check with your insurance company about coverage before your surgery. Some plans need to preauthorize your surgery and your hospital stay. In addition, ask

- If your specific surgery is covered including the length of hospital stay
- Whether aids such as braces, walkers, reachers, and sock-aids (devices to extend your reach) are covered
- If physical therapy is covered in the hospital and when you get home
- If a stay in a transitional care unit/rehabilitation center is covered

Consider writing a health care directive (also known as an advance directive). This document gives legally binding guidance to your family members and health care team about your wishes for medical care in the event you can't communicate. Bring a copy of your health care directive to the hospital when you are admitted and share it with the hospital staff. It is best to develop your health care directive with your attorney. However, legally acceptable forms are available on two websites—www.caringinfo.org and www.aging-withdignity.org/5wishes.html.

Think ahead about the possibility of a blood transfusion. There are three possible choices for a blood donor:

- Yourself
- A specified donor (must have the same blood type)
- A blood bank

If you prefer to use your own blood or that of a specified donor, you must make these arrangements ahead of time. Call your surgeon's office and find out what the procedure is and what blood bank is recommended.

▌ Step 2: Readying Your Home for Your Return

Planning ahead by readying your home can make your return smoother and safer. Put important items within easy reach. You don't want to bend down to get your coffee or reach high overhead for a drinking glass. Put these things on a waist-high countertop or table.

Remove obstacles that pose a tripping hazard. Secure the edges of larger rugs with double-face tape. Remove throw rugs completely. Get rid of or reroute telephone or electric cords that are in your walking path.

You can greatly simplify the demands on your body and back by staying on the first floor of your house during the early part of recovery. If you can, prepare a bedroom and bathroom on the first floor.

Add grab bars in the bathroom to help with getting on and off the toilet and in and out of the bathtub or shower. A handheld showerhead can be helpful in the early part of recovery if it is difficult to reach the shower controls.

Make sure the railings along steps are secure. You should have a well-fitting chair with a firm cushion and arms that is comfortable and easy to get out of. Place the telephone and a small notepad within easy reach of this chair.

When you get home, it will be easiest to wear comfortable, loose-fitting clothing. These garments should be easy to get on and loose enough so that they don't rub or irritate the surgery site. Flat-heeled slip-on shoes (no laces) with firm support (appropriate for walking) will be helpful because you won't need to bend over to put them on. Comfortable, easy-to-don socks are a must (no pantyhose). Your hospital health care team will supply you with dressing aids such as a long-handled shoehorn and sock-aids as needed.

▮ Step 3: Setting Up a Support System

When you first arrive home, it will be difficult if not impossible to perform many household chores. Friends and family members often offer to pitch in, and you can set up a simple schedule so that someone will be there when you need assistance. Consider help with these tasks:

- Shopping for groceries and putting them away (or use an online grocer)
- Caring for your pet (or consider kenneling your dog or cat for a short time)
- Cooking and meal preparation (consider freezing some meals before your surgery or arranging for home delivery of healthy meals)

The early part of your recovery can be emotional and socially stressful. You might feel isolated because you cannot go out easily. It may be hard to adjust to a change in your routine. You can head off depression by lining up support and welcoming visitors. This is actually a better time for visitors than in the hospital. In the hospital, you will be more uncomfortable and tired. Your energy will be needed for learning all you can about caring for your back. Simply ask friends and family to visit you at home when you feel better but may also feel isolated.

If you think it might be necessary, arrange for a stay in a transitional care unit or rehabilitation facility. You can tour these places ahead of time and find one that suits your needs where you will be the most comfortable. Your surgeon's office staff can assist you in making these arrangements. Check ahead of time to make sure your insurance covers your stay.

▮ Step 4: Preparing for Your Hospital Stay

Preparation for your hospital stay begins with packing your suitcase. Label all items with your name. Pack one set of loose-fitting clothes along with appropriate shoes and socks. Pack personal items such as a toothbrush, comb or brush, shaving kit, glasses/contact lenses, and your brace if you were fitted with one before surgery. Bring important documents such as your insurance card, a list of over-the-counter and prescription medications, and your health care directive.

Review any patient information given to you by the surgeon or the hospital. The more you know about the process ahead of time, the more comfortable you will be on the day of surgery.

The Night Before and Morning of Surgery

Your surgeon will have given you specific directions as to when to stop eating and drinking and what medications should be taken the night before and morning of surgery. Heed this advice carefully. It is important to your health and safety.

If a presurgical enema is required, follow the instructions given by the doctor or the doctor's staff. Follow any skin-cleansing instructions carefully.

Prearrange for someone to drive you to the hospital, or surgical center, and home at discharge. If no one is available, use a taxi.

You will be admitted to the hospital on the day of the surgery. After the admission process, you will meet with various members of the surgical team. These include your surgeon, the anesthesiologist (a board-certified anesthesia physician), perhaps a nurse-anesthetist, and the nurses involved with your care. Most spine surgeries are done under general anesthesia, meaning you are "put to sleep" for the duration of the operation. A few procedures are done under local anesthesia, meaning the area of the operation is numbed, but you are not asleep.

Before going to the operating room, most patients are given a sedative medication that makes you drowsy and relaxed. Be sure you ask any final questions before getting this medication. You will wake up in the recovery room where you will be taken care of by special nurses who work only in that area. When you are sufficiently awake you will be taken to your room or, in special cases, to an intensive care unit.

▌ Step 5: Learning the Most in the Hospital

Your Health Care Team

Your hospital care will be provided by different health care professionals including

- The surgeon and his or her staff. These people will meet with you daily after your surgery to assess your progress and generally direct your care. They will decide when you are ready to go home.
- The nurses. They will provide personal care and support and educate you during your hospital stay.

- A social worker or care coordinator. He or she will help you arrange for home care or extra help in your home. If you need placement in a transitional care unit or rehabilitation facility for a short time, a social worker or care coordinator can assist with those plans. Social workers are knowledgeable about community resources and are helpful in figuring out insurance benefits.
- The physical therapists. They will teach you how to get in and out of bed safely, help you begin to walk again after surgery, instruct you in an exercise program, and educate you in proper body mechanics and alignment.
- The occupational therapists. They will teach you safe and energy-saving ways to care for yourself after surgery including how to dress, shower, and bathe. They will familiarize you with aids such as reachers that can ease the performance of everyday tasks. They will teach you how to use proper body alignment during daily life, work, and leisure activities.
- An orthotist. If a brace is ordered by your surgeon, an orthotist will fit you with it and teach you how to use it.
- A dietitian. He or she will make sure your nutritional needs are met during the hospital stay and teach you a diet plan that will foster healing when you get home.

During your hospital stay, make the most of your time with these professionals, listening carefully to what they teach you. Ask questions if something is hard to understand or request written materials.

Understanding Pain Management

You are entitled to proper management of your pain after surgery. If you are comfortable, you will heal better and faster. You are responsible for honestly and clearly communicating your pain level to the nurses and doctor(s). They will respond to the information you give them with appropriate medical intervention.

Pain management begins when you wake up from surgery. Your nurse will ask how you are feeling and how much pain you have. A pain scale from 1 to 10 is often used, with 1 meaning you are having no pain and 10 meaning your pain is the worst possible. These pain management methods may be used during your hospital stay:

- A patient-controlled analgesia (PCA) pump is typically hooked up during surgery and may be continued for up to three days. The PCA allows you to adjust the dose of pain medication directly into your bloodstream by pushing a handheld button.
- Intravenous medications are administered through a vein in your arm.
- Intrathecal (in the fluid around the spinal cord) medications are injected into your spine one time during surgery to alleviate postoperative pain.
- Intramuscular injections are pain medications administered by the nurse by injection (typically into your buttocks).
- Oral medications are pain pills you take by mouth. You will leave the hospital with oral pain medications.

Throughout your hospital stay, diligently monitor your pain level and communicate how you are feeling to your nurses. There are no rewards for toughing it out and being in pain. It only hinders your recovery. Conversely, if you overanalyze your pain, you will become emotionally and physically tense. If you find yourself obsessing about your pain, try distracting yourself with music or the television. Or do a few relaxation exercises.

The Ins and Outs of Your Hospital Stay

Immediately after surgery, you will be taken to a recovery area for a few hours. When your blood pressure and breathing are stable, you will be moved to your assigned bed on the hospital floor.

During the first twenty-four hours after surgery, pain management is important. Communicate your pain needs with the nurses. They will also help you with positioning in bed. You may have a catheter (a thin flexible tube that withdraws urine from the bladder through the urethra) after surgery. The nurses will assist you with it as needed. Your food and drink intake is limited to ice chips. When you are awake, do 10 repetitions of ankle pumps. Rest as much as possible during this time.

During the twenty-four to forty-eight hours after surgery, you will meet with your physical therapist, who will assist you in log rolling to change positions or to sit on the edge of the bed. He or she will also start your exercise program. Regularly perform your deep breathing and coughing exercises (the nurses will remind you) and continue to monitor and communicate your pain level.

You can begin some simple personal care such as washing your face and brushing your teeth while sitting on the edge of the bed. If your bowel activity permits, a clear liquid diet will be started.

In the two to three days after surgery, you will continue to talk with your nurse about pain management. Your activity level will gradually increase to sitting in a chair two times per day and walking short distances with the assistance of the physical therapist or nurse. Initially, you may use a walker when walking for safety reasons.

You will begin to use the bedside commode or bathroom. You might be able to shower with your wound covered. A diet of solid foods will be started.

After the third day, you will continue to progress toward the goals of

- Controlling pain with oral medications
- Getting out of bed and walking safely and independently
- Managing your own personal hygiene
- Tolerating a solid diet

- Being independent in the bathroom (urinating and having bowel movements regularly)
- Keeping a clean and dry incision

Once these goals are met, you are ready for discharge.

You will be discharged when your health care team feels you are ready to go home (or to a transitional care unit). Be sure to ask any questions you might have before you leave (especially about pain management), and be certain you have the contact numbers of personnel if any questions or needs come up when you are at home. Make sure you understand what medications you will be taking and the directions for their use as well as your activity and exercise guidelines. At discharge you are expected to shower, transfer, and reposition yourself, walk independently, and eat a regular diet.

Don't leave the hospital with unanswered questions or incomplete knowledge about your care or condition. Your comfort at discharge will be enhanced if you learn as much as you can during your hospital stay. Your health care team is there to help you. Take advantage of their assistance.

18

The Mind–Body Connection

There is a powerful connection between your body and your mind. Your mind influences your level of pain and suffering through negative or positive thoughts. Believe it or not, this is good news. Once you realize the power your thoughts have over your back pain, you can use this knowledge to your advantage. You can take charge of your thoughts and use them in ways that decrease your pain, speed your healing, and enhance your recovery.

■ Automatic Thinking

Your mind is constantly working. It takes in and evaluates information about things that are happening around you and within you. Most of these thoughts occur outside your awareness and are called automatic thoughts, meaning they are unconscious (you are not immediately aware of them), but they are also very believable. They influence how you feel and how you behave. As you will learn later, they also influence your pain.

Evaluating Your Thoughts

Automatic thoughts are either positive or negative. Positive thoughts reflect reality, help you problem solve, and help you cope with difficulties. By contrast, negative thoughts distort reality, create heavy emotions (such as anxiety, depression, and fear), and increase your pain.

Research shows that when people are under stress, they tend to engage in negative thoughts that are irrational and maladaptive. Having a back problem is stressful. You may have already begun to believe some of these negative automatic thoughts about your back:

- My pain is never going to get better.
- I'm never going to be able to do any of the things I enjoy.
- My pain is getting worse and worse. I am becoming a cripple.
- My life is ruined.

Just reading this list of negative statements creates negative emotions. Automatically repeating these thoughts in your head makes them more and more believable. In reality, if you carefully evaluate these thoughts, they are not true. Negative automatic thinking makes you more nervous, more helpless, and sadder.

Using Automatic Thoughts to Your Benefit

Positive thoughts are rational. They help you cope with your back problem. They lighten the emotional toll of stress and pain. Positive coping thoughts are not false optimism. They are based on the true reality of your situation. They help you focus on the best choices and the best solutions. These coping thoughts lead to the best outcomes:

- I will choose to be optimistic about resolving my back problems.

- I will diligently and persistently seek the best help.
- I will do all I can to help my back heal.

Reviewing this list of optimistic thoughts helps you feel more hopeful. It can also lessen your pain. Using positive automatic thoughts to your benefit is a simple process.

1. Assess your automatic thoughts. Take some time to allow yourself to become aware of the negative thoughts you have about your back and write them down.

2. Refute negative thoughts with positive ones. For each negative thought you discover, think about and write down a positive one. The positive thought should directly counter the negative one. For example, if your negative thought is *I cannot cope with this pain,* counter it with a positive thought such as *I am learning ways to cope with my pain.* Or if you are thinking *I should be better by now,* refute this negative thought with *I am doing the best I can.*

3. Repeatedly review a list of positive thoughts until they become automatic. Repeating the positive thoughts helps solidify them in your mind and makes them more and more believable. They will help you cope and will lead to hope and optimism.

At first, it might be difficult to identify your automatic negative thoughts. Negative feelings will alert you to their presence because negative thinking creates negative emotions.

Think about the negative feelings you are experiencing (or have experienced) about your back pain. These might include fear, sadness, hopelessness, anxiousness, and despair. Next, identify the negative thinking that is causing the emotion. It might be a thought such as *My back is weak and vulnerable to reinjury,* which creates fear. Or, *I am never going to get better,* which creates hopelessness. Or, *I should be better by now,* which creates despair. Once you are aware of the negative feeling and negative thoughts, you can use a coping thought to refute the negative one.

It will take time and practice to change your automatic thoughts. Writing down positive coping thoughts and regularly reviewing them can solidify their presence and their effect. You could even carry a note with a positive thought written on it throughout the day. Hope and optimism are powerful allies in alleviating back pain. Positive thinking is where hope and optimism are born.

Stress

Anyone with a back problem has experienced stress: the stress of having things to do and being too sore to do them, the stress of a sleepless night because of pain, the stress of watching others do the things you enjoy and not being able to participate.

Stress is a physical reaction to a threatening situation or event. When real danger exists, such as a fierce dog chasing you, the stress reaction is helpful. It makes your body ready for action. Unfortunately, the stress reaction can be overused, which causes all sorts of problems.

Your body responds to stress with an increase in blood pressure, an increase in heart rate, faster breathing, and more muscle tension. It is like revving a car engine hard. The problem is that just like running a car engine beyond its designed capabilities will blow up the engine, long-term stress can damage your body. Stress has been linked to several medical problems including headaches, digestive problems, sleeping disorders, and back pain. Stress has been shown to make nearly every medical problem worse and to make surgical procedures more difficult.

Lowering Your Stress Level

Lowering your stress level is an important way to minimize and cope with your back pain. You can directly lessen stress by challenging negative beliefs about your back. Remember that negative thoughts create negative feelings. The sum of these negative feelings is stress. The more negative feelings you have, the more stress you will feel. Fortunately, you can lower your stress by adopting positive beliefs about your back as outlined in the section on automatic thinking.

Another way to lower your stress is by simplifying the demands on you, your time, and your financial resources. Let's face it—the more you have to do, the more stress you feel. Carefully evaluate whether simplifying your life could help relieve stress. Consider whether you can

- Commit less time and energy to stressful relationships
- Ask for or pay for help with house and yard work
- Eliminate the extras that are fun to have but hard to keep up (e.g., a boat, lake home, garden, etc.)
- Let go of volunteer positions at church, at school, or in the community

Combating Stress with Relaxation Training

Relaxation training is an important stress-fighting tool. Relaxation training is not just taking it easy or being a couch potato—it is a specific skill for decreasing stress and muscle tension. It has been shown to effectively combat the physical responses to stress—for example, it can

- Decrease your heart rate
- Lower your blood pressure
- Slow your breathing
- Decrease muscle tension

Deep breathing, mental imagery, and meditation are effective relaxation techniques. They are simple to learn and easy to use.

Deep Breathing

Begin by assuming a comfortable position in a quiet place. You may want to lie on your back or sit in a supportive chair with your feet flat on the floor. Once you are comfortable, you can begin.

1. Take a few moments to review some positive statements about relaxation such as "Relaxation is good for me and for my back" and "I am able to relax."
2. Now inhale deeply through your nose, allowing the air to fill your lungs. Your abdomen will expand or rise as you do.
3. Exhale through your mouth, gently blowing the air out of your lungs.
4. Rather than trying hard to relax or to control what happens, allow the relaxation response to happen on its own.
5. Continue this routine for ten minutes or more.

Like every new skill, relaxation through deep breathing will require practice. Try choosing a regular time to practice and stick with it. After you have effectively learned this technique, you can use it anywhere—for example, when you feel yourself getting tense in rush-hour traffic or when the boss has given you more work than you can get done.

Imagery Training

Another relaxation technique is mental imagery or visualization. The technique is simple—you just picture a pleasant scene or situation. Imagery is a skill you already possess. For example, if you hear the word *vacation,* an image comes to your mind. Imagery training uses your imagination in a specific way to combat stress and tension. Begin by assuming a comfortable position in a quiet place.

1. Imagine a scene that is pleasant and calm. It works best if you imagine a familiar scene.
2. Try to sense the image in many ways. Note what you feel, hear, and smell. Take your time, patiently allowing the scene to fully develop.
3. Now let yourself just be in the scene fully and peacefully. Try to stay with it for at least ten minutes so that you have time to relax and develop the image. Let the scene evolve naturally. Don't control it.
4. End your imagery training session gradually. Don't just stop. Take several deep breaths, inhaling through your nose and exhaling through your mouth. Open your eyes and say to yourself, "I feel relaxed and alert."

Imagery training can be a great tool during stressful medical situations. Instead of focusing on the stressful procedure, imagine a calm scene—for example, if you are anxious about having blood drawn, you can close your eyes and put yourself in a peaceful place.

Imagery and Healing

Imagery can be used to effectively help your body heal from injury or to recover from surgery. It works to activate your body's natural healing abilities. You might try these images:

- Picture your blood bringing important healing nutrients to your pain site and carrying away any damaged cells or tissue.
- Imagine your tight muscles as knots that you slowly loosen so that blood flows freely and carries away tension.
- See your surgery site healing and getting stronger.

Meditation

Meditation can be used to lower stress and promote relaxation. The benefits of meditation include

- Decreased heart rate, blood pressure, and breathing rate
- Decreased muscle tension
- Lowered levels of stress hormones

One simple meditation technique is outlined in Herbert Benson's classic book, *The Relaxation Response.*

1. Sit quietly in a comfortable position with your eyes closed. Relax all of your muscles beginning with your feet and working upward to your face. Keep all your muscles relaxed.
2. Breathe through your nose, becoming aware of each breath. Then begin saying "one" with each exhalation. Continue for ten to twenty minutes.
3. When your thoughts begin to wander, direct yourself back to breathing and repeating "one" with each exhalation.

Other Relaxation Techniques

The relaxation techniques you learned in this chapter are the easiest to learn and use. There are many other relaxation techniques you can try.

Biofeedback training involves placing electrodes on your skin to monitor your physical processes such as heart rate and muscle tension. A monitor provides you with direct feedback on these processes so that you can learn how to control them. Biofeedback is done by trained professionals and involves fairly sophisticated equipment.

Hypnosis is usually performed by a trained medical professional and involves creating a state of focused concentration so that you can relax your mind and body. Hypnosis is not a state of deep sleep or unconsciousness; rather it is a state of relaxed attention.

Guided imagery involves allowing another person to guide you into a state of relaxation. One type of guided imagery is progressive muscle relaxation in which you systematically tighten then relax the muscles throughout your body.

19

Recovering Quickly and Safely After Surgery

Returning home after surgery helps things seem a bit more normal. It feels good to be in a familiar environment, but it can also feel a little scary being on your own. Challenges lie ahead. Knowing what to expect can ease your fears and help you recover quickly and safely.

▮ Expectations

Recovering from surgery is rarely smooth sailing. Most people experience good days and bad. You might be surprised to feel optimistic and hopeful one day and tired and depressed the next. You might even have days when you question if surgery was the right choice. These ups and downs are characteristic of the recovery phase. Expect them. They are normal.

There is no standard recovery time after surgery, since there is such a large variety of surgeries, coupled with different ages and states of general health. During this time, your body is doing a lot of healing. You can help your healing by doing these things:

- Be patient with yourself. Don't get down when you have a bad day. Don't blame yourself if your pain flares up.
- Follow *all* your discharge and recovery instructions.
- Ask for help when you need it.
- If questions arise or if an emergency occurs, have the number for your surgeon's office handy. Don't hesitate to use it if you need to.
- Work to stay optimistic about your recovery. Refute negative thoughts with positive ones.
- Surround yourself with supportive people. This can help fend off feelings of loneliness and isolation.
- Use mental imagery to activate your body's healing abilities by mentally picturing your back getting stronger as it heals.
- Take care of yourself by eating healthy meals, drinking adequate amounts of water, and getting plenty of rest. Follow the list beginning on page 203 and consult a dietitian if you have questions.

■ Controlling Your Pain

Follow the directions for the pain medications you were given when you left the hospital. Don't hesitate to use these medications appropriately if you are in pain. That is what they are for.

Besides taking pain medication, there are several other things you can do to help control and lessen your pain. Heat or cold can be used. Try both, and stick with the one that is most effective for you. A cold pack or heating pad can be applied to the painful area for ten to twenty minutes, but be sure to avoid the surgical site. Do not sleep with a heating pad because it creates a burn risk.

You can help control your pain by carefully choosing how you sit or lie. Do not sit for more than thirty minutes before getting up to stretch or taking a brief walking break. Do not sit on a chair or couch that forces you to sit in a slouched position. Sit in a sturdy chair that supports your back and allows you to sit with your feet on the floor. Use a lumbar support if that helps.

If you are becoming overfocused on your pain (if you are thinking and/or worrying about it most of the time), try distracting yourself. Rent a good movie or listen to your favorite music. Use mental imagery to occupy your mind with a pleasant scene. Invite a friend or family member over for a visit.

Relaxation training can also be used to control pain. Use deep breathing and/or mental imagery. See Chapter 18 for various mental relaxation techniques. You can also add a few drops of scented oil to a damp washcloth, then fold it and place it over your closed eyes as you inhale the relaxing scent.

A final strategy for pain control is drawing on the emotional support of friends and family members who care about you. Sharing your ups and downs with a trusted ally can help you feel supported and cared for.

▌ Self-Care

Your recovery time will afford you many opportunities to practice self-care. Follow all the instructions given to you in the hospital. Some of them may seem trivial, but every one of them is designed to give you the safest and quickest recovery. If you stopped smoking before or during your hospital stay, don't start up now. Your body is using its resources to heal from surgery. Smoking hinders your body's healing capacity.

A critical part of self-care is following the limitations given to you in the hospital. Generally a 5-pound lifting limit is the norm after spine surgery. In addition, you should avoid twisting your spine to turn. Turn with your whole body instead. Avoid excess pulling, pushing, and reaching. Practice proper technique when picking up objects, getting in and out of the car, and bending or lifting.

Part of self-care is emotional self-care. Practice being gentle and patient with yourself. You will benefit most from positive and affirmative self-talk. You are not going to do your recovery perfectly. Maybe you will mistakenly overdo it and have a pain flare-up. Rather than shaming and blaming yourself, view it as a learning opportunity. Use what you learn to avoid making the same mistake again.

Sexual activity after back surgery might require some adaptations. It is best for you to have your back supported on the bed—the missionary position if you are female, the female superior position if you are male. Initially, you should assume a more passive role and your partner the more active role. As your back heals, you can gradually resume a more active role. Avoid "acrobatic" maneuvers.

▌ Increasing Your Activity Level

One word defines how to increase your activity level: *gradually*. Your surgeon sent you home with some specific activity limitations. Follow them diligently. In addition, pace yourself as you resume activities. Try them for a defined amount of time, then gradually increase the time length. Give yourself plenty of breaks, and don't persist in one position or activity for too long. For example, if you are going to sit down at the computer, start with a ten-minute session. Get up and give yourself a break, or move on to a different activity. The next time, try a fifteen-minute session, and gradually build up from there.

▌ Walking Program

Your surgeon probably gave you instructions for a walking program. If not, ask if it is okay to use the one outlined here. Don't start without first checking with your surgeon. Walking is not appropriate for some people after surgery. An alternative activity might be recommended such as swimming or stationary bicycling.

▌ Walking Precautions ▌

1. Gradually increase how far you walk and how fast you walk.
2. Avoid steep hills, ice, grass, and other uneven surfaces. A mall, grocery store, fitness center, or community center are good alternative places to walk.
3. If it is very hot, walk in the morning and the evening when it is cooler.
4. Be sure you do not bend forward at the waist while you walk.
5. Listen to your body. You should breathe comfortably as you walk. If you become breathless, slow down. Pay attention to your pain level. If your pain intensifies as you walk, slow down for a while. If slowing down doesn't help, stop for this session and try again later in the day or the next day.
6. Wear a well-cushioned shoe that will absorb shock and provide protection for your healing back. Comfortable, loose clothing allows you to move freely. Consider dressing in layers. As you heat up, take a layer off; if you cool down, put it back on.
7. Rest between walks. You might lie on your back with pillows under your knees. Use ice or heat on your back as seems helpful.
8. If one walk is enough on some days, skip the second walk.

How Much, How Often, How Fast

Frequency is how often you walk. We recommend two short walks each day, five days per week. Two walks per day gets you out of the house and into the larger world, which is good for your mental outlook. A brief walk is also easier on your healing back than a longer walk. Resting between brief walks gives your muscles time to recover.

Duration is how long you walk. Five to ten minutes is long enough when you are starting out. People with good general health can usually work up to walks of three to five miles per day.

Intensity is how fast you walk. During this recovery phase, you should always walk at a comfortable pace. Don't worry about pushing it. Walk so that you can breathe comfortably. You should not be breathless.

▮ Safely Performing Daily Activities

As you start to resume your normal life, you will find there are a lot of things you need to do differently.

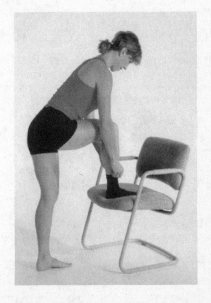

1. Dressing. Instead of bending over to put your socks on, use a sock-aid or put your foot on a chair and bend forward from the hips (not from the trunk; your back should be straight, not rounded). Sit down to put on your pants, keeping a straight spine as you do. A long-handled shoehorn can help with putting on shoes. Elastic laces or Velcro closures make it easier to put your shoes on and take them off.

2. Showering and bathing. Getting in and out of the bathtub can seem like a formidable task after back surgery. You can try using a tub bench to sit on. A handheld showerhead makes it easier to reach. Showers can be easier to manage.

3. Bending and lifting. If you drop an object or need to pick something up from the floor, use a reacher to minimize bending or try the golfer's lift.

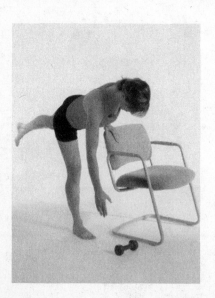

Golfer's Lift Place one hand on a firm surface, then let one leg go back in the air as you reach toward the floor. This keeps your back straight as you bend.

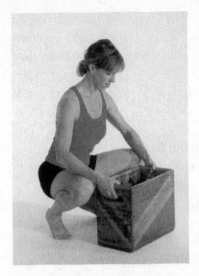
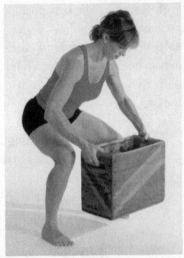

Two-Leg Lift Position your feet a little wider than your shoulders. Bend your knees, but keep your back straight. Bring the object you are lifting as close to you as possible (but do not allow your chest to slump). Now stand up by straightening your legs.

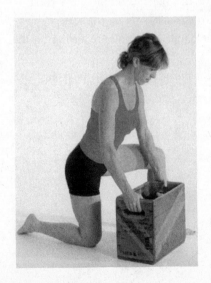

Half-Kneel Lift This lift works well for lifting groceries or suitcases. Place one foot in front of the other. Keeping your back straight, bend at the knees to a half-kneeling position. Grasp the object you are lifting and push up through both legs to standing. Be sure to keep your trunk straight as you come up.

4. Sleeping. The best positions for sleeping are usually lying on your back (with pillows under your knees if that is more comfortable) or lying on your side with a pillow between your knees (and maybe one at your chest to hug).

5. Riding in a car. Use this technique for getting in and out of the car:

▮ Getting in the Car ▮

- Push the seat back as far as it will go.
- Position yourself with your back to the seat.
- Keeping your back straight, lower yourself to the seat.
- Now turn your whole body, lifting your legs into the car.

After riding for thirty minutes, try taking a break. Stop and stretch or take a short walk.

▮ Getting Out of the Car ▮

- Slide closer to the driver's seat.
- Turn your body toward the outside of the car—rotating your buttocks until your legs are lying on the seat.
- Push forward with your hands until you are sitting on the edge of the seat.
- Use the back of the seat and dashboard to push up to a standing position.

20

How Do I Get Back to Work?

You and your doctor will decide how and when you return to work. If you have a work-related injury and/or if there is some question as to whether you can return to your usual job, this is a more complicated matter. In this case, the coordinated involvement of your doctor, your employer, workers' compensation officials, lawyers, and perhaps others is required. There is an enormous variation depending on age, health, and type of surgery.

■ Returning to Work with or without Restrictions

Your doctor may set limits about what you can do at work and/or how long you can do it. Your doctor might place restrictions on how much you can lift, how long you can stand or sit, and how often you can bend or lift. You might start back to work on a part-time basis. Or you and your doctor may decide that you are ready to return to work full-time and to carry out your full-time job duties. You might return to your previous job but with appropriate medical restrictions.

Changing Jobs

A back problem might prevent you from returning to your previous job. In this case, you might want to pursue vocational rehabilitation to learn a new job within your medical restrictions.

Returning to Work Is Prohibited

Occasionally but very rarely the doctor and back patient may decide together that returning to work is not an option. This is most likely if you are advanced in age and have had multiple back surgeries with loss of nerve function and resultant medical restriction. In this case, permanent disability would be recommended.

▌ Vocational Rehabilitation and Work Hardening

Your doctor may consider referring you to vocational rehabilitation or work hardening. Vocational rehabilitation is a service that specializes in helping injured workers return to work. Vocational rehabilitation therapists can help you negotiate your return to your old job. Or if that is not possible, they can help you learn what jobs are available and the qualifications for those jobs. They can also help you understand your limitations and the types of jobs most suitable for your medical restrictions.

Work hardening is a structured rehabilitation program that uses real or simulated work activities to restore physical and vocational function. Work hardening involves an analysis of the physical demands of your job followed by a graduated strengthening program to train and recondition your body for return to work. This program is particularly helpful if you have a physically demanding job and/or if you have been out of the workforce for quite some time.

▌ Preparing to Return to Work

The transition back to work is more likely to go smoothly if you are well prepared.

- *Be mentally prepared.* You can mentally prepare for returning to work by deliberately spending time picturing a successful return to work in your mind. This will build positive expectations and help alleviate the fear and anxiety that is generated by anticipating a negative experience.
- *Be realistic.* Realistically, the transition back to work will probably have some ups and downs. It will take some time for your body to adjust to the demands placed on it at work.
- *Be prepared for flare-ups.* You might experience a flare-up in your back pain as you adjust to the different physical demands at work. You can cope with these episodes by trying over-the-counter medications (especially the NSAIDs such as Advil and Alleve), using heat or ice (whichever is more beneficial), and doing your physical therapy exercise program (if you have been given one). You can also follow the self-care guidelines in Chapter 8.

▌ Working Smart

Working smart is one of the best ways to prevent flare-ups or reinjury. Three important parts of working smart are using good body mechanics, using good posture, and pacing.

Use Good Body Mechanics

Good body mechanics means using your body—and especially your back—in the safest manner. Avoid twisting at the trunk. Twisting is particularly stressful to the spine. As much as possible, avoid repetitive bending. When you do bend, use your legs instead of your back. Bend from the knees, not from the waist. Another safe way to bend is the golfer's lift (page 228).

Lifting is another important part of good body mechanics. Two useful methods of lifting are the two-leg lift and the half-kneel lift (page 229).

Use Good Posture

Sitting can be a stressful position for your back. Good sitting posture begins with selecting a good chair. As much as possible, choose a firm chair that supports your back. Avoid soft chairs that force you to slump.

Good Sitting Posture

Good sitting posture means

- The S curve of the spine is maintained
- Your ears, shoulders, and hips should line up to ensure that your trunk remains straight
- Using a lumbar cushion, if needed, to support the lower back

Good Standing Posture

Good standing posture places the body in balanced upright alignment. There is minimal muscle effort, and the body is comfortable, not strained. Good standing posture means

- Having knees that are relaxed and relatively straight but not locked
- Having a mild curve in your lower back
- The ears, shoulders, hips, and knees are aligned in side view
- Your feet are shoulder width apart, and your weight is balanced evenly between your two legs

One variation on good standing posture is to place the heel of one foot next to the arch of the other foot. Your weight should remain balanced between the two legs.

Pacing

Pacing involves taking regular breaks so that your spine isn't in the same position for too long. It also involves varying your activities so that your back gets a break from doing the same thing over and over again. For example, if your job requires a lot of sitting, take breaks every twenty to thirty minutes to stand up and walk around. Or if you do a lot of repetitive bending, take regular breaks to extend your trunk (bend it backward).

■ Returning to the Office

If you are returning to an office job, you can help your transition back to work by setting up your desk, chair, and computer properly.

Chair

Your chair is the most important piece of equipment in your office. It should be comfortable and have the following characteristics:

- Adjustable height
- Lumbar support
- A good backrest that is wide enough to support your shoulders
- A seat that allows 1 to 4 inches of space between the edge of the chair and your knees.
- A seat with a curved front edge

Desk

Your desk should be big enough for heavily used items so that you don't have to constantly stretch, twist, and turn to get what you need.

Computer

The monitor should be positioned to minimize stress to the neck and back. It should be

- Positioned so that the screen is slightly below eye level
- About 20 to 24 inches away from you
- Cleaned regularly and positioned to minimize glare

The keyboard should be positioned to allow for upper arm relaxation. Your upper arms should rest comfortably at your sides with your forearms at a right angle to the upper arms.

21

Keeping Your Back Healthy and Strong

Keeping your back healthy and strong can help minimize or maybe even alleviate your back pain. But a strong and healthy back doesn't just happen. It has to be a deliberate goal that you work toward steadily. These are the key ingredients for a strong and healthy back:

1. A balanced exercise program that includes
   - *A daily stretching program*
   - *Strength training two to three times per week*
   - *Aerobic exercise five to seven times per week*
   - *Being active through safe recreational activity*
2. Sensible eating, which includes
   - *Losing weight (if necessary) and maintaining a healthy weight*
   - *Healthy eating (by following the Mayo Clinic Pyramid on page 269)*
3. No smoking

■ The Stretching Program

Stretching is essential to a healthy back. Stretching promotes muscle and spine flexibility, which in turn makes movement easier and less stressful for the back. The following six stretches should be done on a daily basis. Some people feel best if they do them first thing in the morning. They are also a great way to warm up your body before walking, swimming, or doing other aerobic exercise.

Stretching should always be done gently—you should feel a slight pull in the muscle being stretched, but it should never hurt. If a stretch irritates your back, make sure you are not doing it too aggressively. If doing the stretch gently is still painful for your back, skip that stretch entirely.

The Stretching Exercises

Hamstring Stretch Lie on your back with your left leg bent. Grab behind your right knee with both hands and straighten your right leg. Feel a gentle pull along the back of your right leg (in your hamstring muscles). Hold the stretch for 20 seconds. Repeat on the opposite side. Do this stretch 3 times on one leg, then 3 times on the other leg.

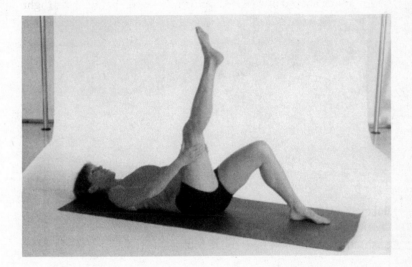

Knee to Chest Lying on your back, bring your right knee up to your chest. Grab behind the right knee with both hands to assist the movement. Hold this position for 10 seconds. Repeat on the opposite side. Do this stretch 5 times on each side, alternating between right and left.

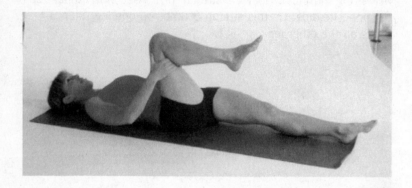

Double Knee to Chest Lying on your back, bring both knees up to your chest, holding behind the knees with your hands. Hold this position for 10 seconds. Repeat 5 times.

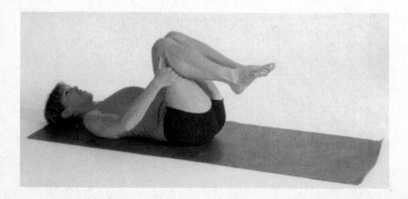

Hip Flexor Stretch In a half-kneeling position, tighten your abdominal muscles. Keeping your trunk erect, move it forward so that you are increasing the bend in the right knee. You will feel a gentle stretch along the front of the left hip. Hold the stretch for 20 seconds. Repeat on the opposite side. Do the stretch 3 times on one side, then 3 times on the other side.

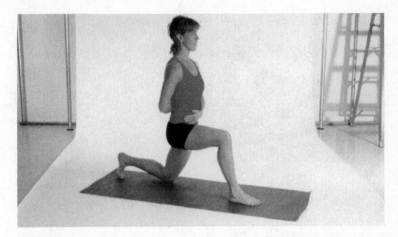

Press-Up Start by lying flat on your stomach with your palms down next to your shoulders. Now press your chest up by straightening your elbows. Keep your hips on the floor. Hold this position for 10 seconds. Repeat 5 times.

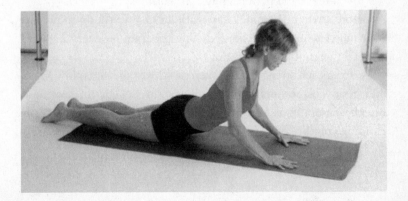

Piriformis Stretch Lying on your back, bring your right knee toward your left shoulder, using your left hand to pull the right knee up and across. You should feel a stretch in your right buttock. Hold the stretch for 20 seconds. Repeat on the opposite side. Do the stretch 3 times on each side.

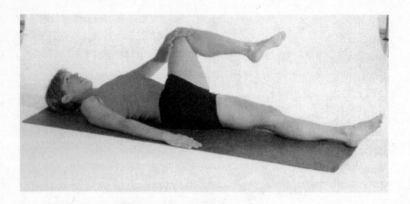

▪ The Strengthening Program

Strength training helps build strong muscles to support your back and prevent injury. Strong muscles lessen the stress on your spine when you move and perform physical work.

Before strength training, start with an easy warm-up to prepare your muscles for work. The stretching program on pages 238–241 is a great warm-up routine.

Perform each strengthening exercise slowly and smoothly. Maintain good posture and good alignment throughout each exercise. Breathe naturally as you strength train. Never hold your breath. Holding your breath can dangerously elevate your blood pressure.

How Much, How Often

Strength training should be done 2 to 3 times per week with at least 1 day between strength training sessions to allow your muscles time to recover.

Each time you perform a strengthening exercise, it counts as a repetition (or rep). To begin, try doing 8 reps of each exercise. The last rep should be difficult to complete, and you should feel some muscle fatigue. If you can't do 8 repetitions, do as many as you can. If you can easily do 8 reps, try 10. If doing 10 reps is easy, try 12. When doing 12 reps is easy, you are ready to move on to the next level.

The strength training program for a strong and healthy back has three levels. Begin with the exercises in level 1. As they become easy, progress to level 2 and then level 3. The exercises at each level are designed to strengthen the back and abdominal muscles as well as some key muscles in the hips and legs.

A set consists of 8 to 12 reps of the same exercise. If completing 1 set of an exercise is too easy, you can try doing 2 sets the next time around. It is okay to do 1 to 3 sets of any exercise. Make sure to gradually increase the number of reps and sets to prevent injury and/or exhaustion. Here is a summary of the back strength training program:

Frequency: 2 to 3 times per week, but not 2 days in a row
Reps: 8 to 12 for each exercise
Sets: at least 1 and up to 3 sets of each exercise
Levels: progressing from level 1 to level 2 to level 3

The Strengthening Exercises

Level 1: The Balanced Strengthening Program
You will need an exercise ball and perhaps an ankle weight (available at sporting goods stores and in the sports department of major retail stores).

1. Abdominal Curl

- *Lie on your back with your knees bent and your feet flat on the floor.*
- *Tighten your abdominal muscles and flatten your back against the floor.*
- *Maintain a flattened back throughout the entire exercise.*
- *Interlace your fingers behind your neck.*
- *Slowly lift your shoulders off the floor, hold, then slowly lower your shoulders to the floor. (Be careful not to "crank" on your neck.) Feel the work primarily along the upper portion of your abs, above the waist.*
- *Complete 8 to 12 reps.*

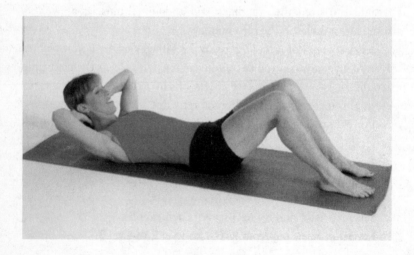

2. Diagonal Abdominal Curl

- *Lie on your back with your knees bent and your feet flat on the floor.*
- *Tighten your abdominal muscles and flatten your back against the floor.*
- *Interlace you fingers behind your neck.*
- *Slowly lift your left shoulder toward your right knee, hold, then slowly lower the left shoulder to the floor.*
- *Complete 8 to 12 reps, alternating right and left.*

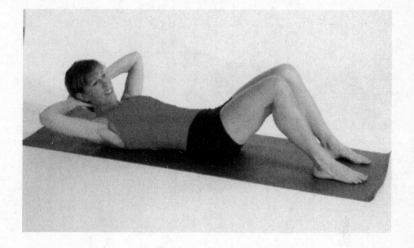

3. Two-Leg Bridging

- *Lie on your back with your knees bent and your feet flat on the floor. Your arms should rest at your sides on the floor.*
- *Tighten your buttock muscles by squeezing your "cheeks" together.*
- *Slowly lift your buttocks so that your knees, hips, and shoulders are aligned. Hold, then slowly lower.*
- *Complete 8 to 12 reps.*

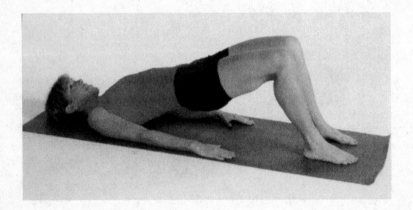

4. Side-Lying Leg Lift

- *Lie on your right side with your head, shoulders, and hips aligned.*
- *Head rests on your extended right arm for alignment.*
- *For balance, put your left hand, palm side down, in front of you.*
- *Lift your left leg slowly, hold, then slowly lower it.*
- *You should feel the muscles working along the outside of your left hip and leg.*
- *Do 8 to 12 reps, then repeat on the other side.*

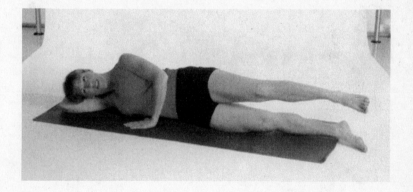

5. All Fours Arm and Leg Lift

- *Start on all fours on the floor.*
- *Make your trunk as flat as a table top (it should not be rounded or arched), then tighten your abdominal muscles.*
- *Keep the trunk "flat" while slowly lifting your right arm and left leg. Hold, then slowly lower the arm and leg.*
- *Complete 8 to 12 repetitions, then repeat with the opposite arm and leg.*

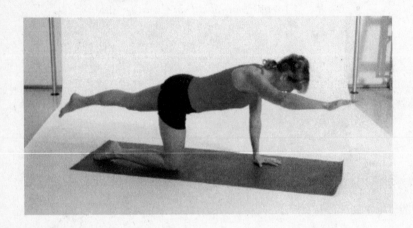

6. Leg Extension on an Exercise Ball

- *Sit on an exercise ball with your hips and knees at a right angle.*
- *Straighten or extend one leg.*
- *Add weights to your ankle as the exercise gets easier.*
- *Complete 8 to 12 repetitions, then repeat with the opposite leg.*

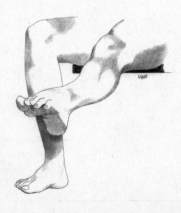

Level 2: The Balanced Strengthening Program

For this level you will need two small dumbbells (3–5 pounds each) and 2–3-pound ankle weights from a weight-lifting set. You will also need an exercise ball. Dumbbells, ankle weights, and exercise balls are available at sporting goods stores and major retail stores.

1. Abdominal Curl with Weights

- *Lie on your back with your knees bent and your feet flat on the floor.*
- *Hold a small dumbbell in each hand and cross them over your chest.*
- *Tighten your abdominal muscles and flatten your back against the floor.*
- *Slowly lift your shoulders off the floor, hold, then slowly lower your shoulders to the floor.*
- *Complete 8 to 12 reps.*

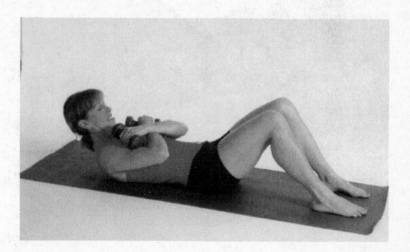

2. Diagonal Abdominal Curl with Weights

- *Lie on your back with your knees bent and your feet flat on the floor.*
- *Hold a small dumbbell in each hand and cross them over your chest.*
- *Tighten your abdominal muscles and flatten your back against the floor.*
- *Slowly lift your left shoulder toward your right knee, hold, then slowly lower the left shoulder to the floor.*
- *Complete 8 to 12 reps, alternating right and left.*

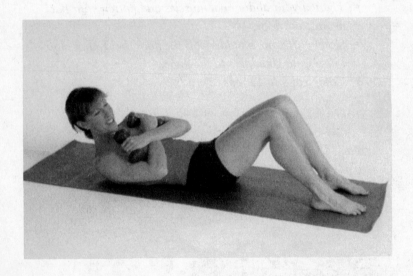

3. One-Leg Bridging

- *Lie on your back with your knees bent and your feet flat on the floor. Your arms should rest at your sides on the floor.*
- *Straighten your right leg so that both knees are parallel.*
- *Tighten your buttock muscles by squeezing your "cheeks" together.*
- *Slowly lift your buttocks so that your knees, hips, and shoulders are aligned. Hold, then slowly lower.*
- *Complete 8 to 12 reps, then repeat on the other side.*

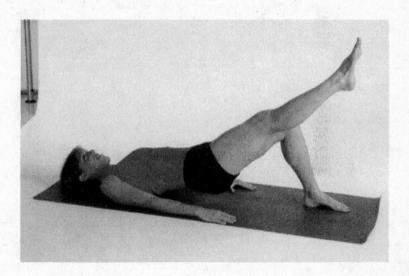

4. Side-Lying Leg Lift with Rotation

- *Lie on your right side with your head, shoulders, and hips aligned.*
- *Head rests on your extended right arm for alignment.*
- *For balance, put your left hand, palm side down, in front of you.*
- *Bend and lift your left leg slowly while rolling or rotating the leg out. Hold, then slowly lower it.*
- *You should feel the muscles working along the outside of your left hip and leg.*
- *Do 8 to 12 reps, then repeat on the other side.*

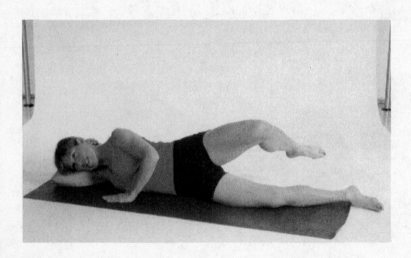

5. Arm Lift on an Exercise Ball

- *Lie over the exercise ball with your palms flat on the floor and your toes touching the ground.*
- *Tighten your abdominal muscles.*
- *Slowly lift your left arm, hold, then slowly lower it. Keep your trunk as steady as you can.*
- *Complete 8 to 12 repetitions, then repeat with the right arm.*

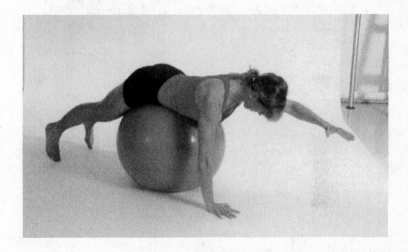

6. Two-Leg Squat with an Exercise Ball

- *Stand with your feet shoulder width apart and lean against the exercise ball (the exercise ball rests on the wall).*
- *Slowly let your knees bend so that your knees are over your toes. Hold, then slowly straighten your knees.*
- *Complete 8 to 12 repetitions.*

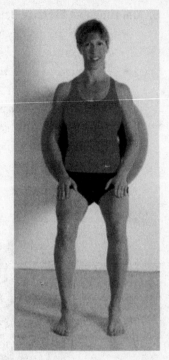

Level 3: The Balanced Strengthening Program

This level requires the use of an exercise ball, a 2- to 3-foot piece of an exercise band, and an ankle weight (available at sporting goods stores and major retail stores).

1. Abdominal Curls on an Exercise Ball

- *Start by sitting on an exercise ball, then roll down it until your back is resting on the ball.*
- *Tighten your abdominal muscles and keep them tight throughout the exercise.*
- *Interlace your fingers behind your neck.*
- *Slowly curl your head, neck, and shoulders up, feeling the abdominal muscles work. Hold, then slowly lower your head, neck, and shoulders.*
- *Complete 8 to 12 repetitions.*

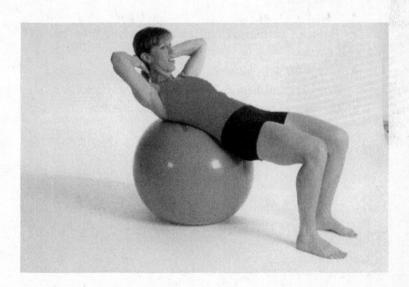

2. Diagonal Abdominal Curl on an Exercise Ball

- *Start by sitting on an exercise ball, then roll down it until your back is resting on the ball.*
- *Tighten your abdominal muscles and keep them tight throughout the exercise.*
- *Interlace your fingers behind your neck.*
- *Slowly bring your left shoulder toward your right knee. Hold, then slowly lower.*
- *Complete 8 to 12 repetitions.*

3. One-Leg Bridging with Ankle Weights

- *Wrap a weight (2 to 3 pounds to start with) around your right ankle.*
- *Lie on your back with your knees bent and your feet flat on the floor. Your arms should rest at your sides on the floor.*
- *Straighten your right leg so that both knees are parallel.*
- *Tighten your buttock muscles by squeezing your "cheeks" together.*
- *Slowly lift your buttocks so that your knees, hips, and shoulders are aligned. Hold, then slowly lower.*
- *Complete 8 to 12 reps, then repeat on the other side. Add more weight as the exercise gets easier.*

4. Side-Lying Leg Rotation with an Exercise Band

- *Lie on your right side with your knees bent and an exercise band tied fairly tightly around your knees.*
- *For balance, put your left hand, palm side down, in front of you.*
- *Roll or rotate your left knee out against the resistance of the tubing, hold, then slowly lower it.*
- *You should feel the muscles working along the outside of your left hip and leg.*
- *Do 8 to 12 reps, then repeat on the other side.*

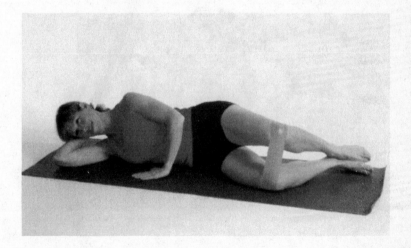

5. Leg Lifts on an Exercise Ball

- *Lie over the exercise ball with your palms flat on the floor and your toes touching the ground.*
- *Tighten your abdominal muscles.*
- *Slowly lift your right leg off the floor, hold, then slowly lower it.*
- *Complete 8 to 12 repetitions, then repeat with the left leg.*

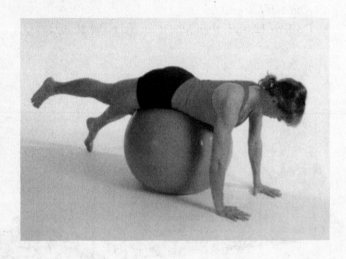

6. One Leg Squat with an Exercise Ball

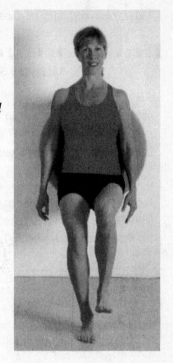

- *Stand on your right leg and lean against an exercise ball (the exercise ball rests on the wall).*
- *Slowly let your left knee bend so that it is over your toes. Hold, then slowly straighten your knee.*
- *Complete 8 to 12 repetitions, then repeat on the other side.*

Here is a summary of the balanced strengthening program:

■■
THE BALANCED STRENGTHENING PROGRAM

	Level 1	Level 2	Level 3
Abdominals	Abdominal Curl	Abdominal Curl with Dumbbells	Abdominal Curl on an Exercise Ball
Diagonal Abdominals (Obliques)	Diagonal Abdominal Curl	Diagonal Abdominal Curl with Weights	Diagonal Abdominal Curl on an Exercise Ball
Buttocks Muscles	Two-Leg Bridging	One-Leg Bridging	One-Leg Bridging with Ankle Weights
Hip Abductors	Side-Lying Leg Lift	Side-Lying Leg Lift with Rotation	Side-Lying Leg Rotation with an Exercise Band
Back Muscles	All-Fours Arm and Leg Lift	Arm Lift on an Exercise Ball	Leg Lift on an Exercise Ball
Thigh Muscles	Leg Extension on an Exercise Ball	Two-Leg Squat with an Exercise Ball	One-Leg Squat with an Exercise Ball

■ Aerobic Exercise

Aerobic exercise is the kind of exercise that gets your heart pumping and increases your oxygen uptake. Aerobic activities include walking, swimming, and running. Aerobic exercise promotes cardiovascular fitness—it makes your heart and circulatory system healthier. It is an absolutely essential part of overall fitness and health. It can help you live longer and healthier and can help you manage or prevent many chronic health conditions. According to the MayoClinic.com website, aerobic exercise

- Reduces your risk for coronary artery disease
- Reduces your risk for developing high blood pressure
- Improves your cholesterol levels
- Reduces your risk for stroke
- Reduces your risk for developing some types of cancer including breast, colon, prostate, and endometrial cancer
- Reduces your risk for developing Type II diabetes
- Wards off viral illness by assisting in activating your immune system and preparing it to fight off infection
- Boosts mood and energy
- Alleviates depression and anxiety
- Reduces back pain and produces significant metabolic changes including elevation of endorphins, which are morphine-like compounds that reduce pain

Walking: The Ideal Aerobic Exercise

Walking is the ideal aerobic exercise because it is easy to do and inexpensive. It requires only two things: a properly fitting pair of shoes and a pedometer. With those two things in place, you are ready to hit the pavement (or the indoor mall or treadmill) and start getting in shape. Try to walk a minimum of five days per week.

What is a pedometer and how do you find one?

A pedometer is a small battery-run device that senses motion. It attaches to your waistband and counts the number of steps you take as you walk and move. It doesn't matter when or how you step. You might be on a walk. You might be walking across the parking lot at work. You might be chasing your toddler around the yard. The pedometer counts all these steps equally and gives you a grand total at the end of the day.

Pedometers are available at sporting goods stores as well as major retail stores. They range in price from $4 to $55 In general, the lower-price models are less reliable and less durable.

Counting Steps

For improved health a good goal is to accumulate 10,000 steps in a day (approximately 2,000 steps=1 mile). If your goal is to boost weight loss, shoot for 12,000 to 15,000 steps per day. If you are at a healthy weight, add 3,000 steps (approximately 1½ miles) to your baseline (the average number of your present daily steps). Here are some simple strategies for increasing the number of steps you take in a day:

- When grocery shopping, go up and down all the aisles.
- Return your shopping cart to the store.
- Park farther away from your destination.
- Take the stairs instead of the elevator.
- When walking the dog, add a few extra blocks.
- Walk the halls at work during lunch and coffee breaks.
- During television commercial breaks, walk in place.

Getting to Your Goal

It is very important to gradually increase the number of steps you take in a day. But before you start, you need to know your steps baseline.

1. Place your pedometer on your waistband near your hip bone.
2. For three days, simply follow your usual routine.
3. At the end of the day, record the number of steps you have accumulated.
4. For every ten minutes of strength training you do, add 1,000 steps.

5. Find the average for those three days by adding together the total from each day and dividing by 3. That is your steps baseline.

Now, each day for a week, try doing 500 steps (approximately ¼ mile) more than your baseline. If your baseline was 3,000 steps, try doing 3,500 steps each day. The next week, try doing 500 more each day—going from 3,500 per day to 4,000 per day. In six weeks, you will have added 3,000 steps. Keep going at this rate until you reach your goal: either 10,000 steps per day for improved health or 12,000 to 15,000 steps for improved health and weight loss.

High-Quality Steps for Better Health

Accumulating 10,000 or more steps is a great way to improve your health. You can give your health and fitness an even greater boost by making sure that five times per week you accumulate steps through vigorous exercise. For example, you might try going on a scheduled walk for thirty to forty-five minutes in which you maintain a vigorous pace. But you don't necessarily have to walk. You can substitute with thirty to forty-five minutes of vigorous housework or yard work as long as you keep moving rather quickly the entire time and are doing moderately physically challenging tasks. Washing and drying dishes won't do. Here is a list of moderately vigorous house and yard chores:

- Sweeping
- Vacuuming
- Picking up, carrying in, and quickly unloading groceries
- Gardening
- Washing windows
- Raking
- Mowing with a push mower
- Shoveling snow

Here is a summary of the pedometer walking program:

1. Use a pedometer to count the number of steps you take in a day.
2. Set a goal of averaging 10,000 steps per day.
3. Work toward reaching that goal gradually by adding an average of 500 steps per day for a week.
4. Five times each week, accumulate thirty to forty-five minutes of steps through moderately vigorous activity.

Other Types of Aerobic Exercise

If walking isn't your cup of tea, you can try swimming, running, or stationary biking. Your goal is to do these activities no less than five times per week for thirty to forty-five minutes at a time in a moderately vigorous manner. It is okay to mix and match—for example, walking three times per week and swimming twice.

Swimming

Swimming is generally an excellent form of exercise for back problems. The buoyancy of the water helps "unweight" your spine while the resistance of the water forces you to move slowly and smoothly.

If you are quite out of shape or if your ability to move is limited by back pain, you can start by simply walking in the pool and gently moving your arms and legs in the water. Another option is a water aerobics class from a certified instructor. Classes are often offered at YMCAs, community pools, and health clubs.

Swimming laps is also great exercise, as long as you can do it without increased pain. Strokes done on your stomach, such as the breaststroke and crawl, cause your back to arch or extend, which can be irritating to some back problems. The butterfly stroke requires both flexing and extending and is therefore quite stressful to the spine. The least stressful strokes are the backstroke and sidestroke.

Running

Running is faster and more intense than walking. The impact of your feet hitting the ground can aggravate back problems. Some important tips for minimizing the impact forces of running are

1. Buy good running shoes. Good shoes will support your feet and absorb shock, minimizing the stress that is transmitted to your back. A reputable running store (not a department store or general sporting goods store) is the best place to purchase running shoes. Change your shoes every 400 to 500 miles, since they lose their ability to absorb shock with extended use.
2. Run on soft, flat, smooth surfaces. Running on a flat, smooth trail is easier on your spine than running on concrete or asphalt. The softer surface means there is less jarring at impact. Running uphill puts your spine in flexion, which may be aggravating to some back problems. Running downhill increases impact force and puts your spine in extension, which may aggravate some back problems.

Biking or Stationary Biking

Biking is a great way to strengthen your legs and get good aerobic exercise. The greatest risk to your back with bike riding is having it hunched forward or flexed for long stretches of time. This can be remedied in several ways. Try lowering the seat and raising the handlebars. This will put your spine in a more upright position. Mountain bikes typically allow a more upright trunk than road bikes, so riding a mountain bike might aggravate your back less. A qualified technician at a good bike shop can check the fit of your bike and make adjustments as necessary.

If you are biking outdoors, stick with flatter rides. Riding uphill causes you to flex your trunk and spine and to strain more, which might aggravate your back. If you are mountain biking, avoid paths that are treacherous enough to cause spills or that have ruts and other rough spots, which might cause jarring to your body and back. In general, you want a ride that is smooth and steady, not one that is rough and hard.

■ Making Recreational Sports and Activities Safe

We hope you're getting the message that it is important to get moving and be active. Participating in recreational sports and activities is a fun way to do that. You might have to modify how you play the game in order to keep your back as safe as possible.

Racquet Sports

Racquet sports include racquetball, tennis, and squash. The risk in these sports comes from twisting, reaching, and lunging. You can minimize the stress to your back during racquet sports by

1. Adjusting your shots. The serve, overhead shot, and backhand are the most likely to irritate a back problem. Work to avoid hyperextending your back and excessively twisting your trunk. See a professional instructor for help if needed.
2. Not lunging at hard-to-reach shots. This can aggravate your back. Learn to let them go.
3. Trying a back brace. A back brace can support and protect your back while limiting excess motion.

Weight Lifting

Lifting weights puts a great amount of pressure on your spine. Don't do this without carefully consulting your spine doctor. The amount of stress depends on the type and intensity of weight lifting you do. These tips can help make weight lifting safer:

1. Decrease the amount of weight you lift and increase the number of repetitions. This decreases the stress to your back but still allows you to get a good workout. Always lift within your ability. Excess straining can cause or irritate back problems.
2. Use good technique. A trained professional such as a personal trainer, physical therapist, or athletic trainer can teach you proper, safe weight-lifting technique. Good technique typically breaks down when you are tired at the end of a workout or when you are lifting too much weight. Use a mirror to self-monitor your technique.
3. Use a weight-lifting belt. A weight-lifting belt (available at sporting goods stores) supports your lower back.
4. Choose movements that are easiest on your back. Focus on a routine that doesn't put excess stress on your back. Consult with a personal trainer or physical therapist to find the proper exercises for you. If a weight-lifting exercise hurts your back, stop doing it.

Golf

The golf swing uses a twisting motion that puts significant stress on your back. That is why many professional golfers have back problems. Some helpful tips for minimizing the stress on your back during golf include

1. Warming up and stretching. Many golfers forget to warm up and stretch before swinging the club. Warming up is a great way to prepare your body and your back for the demands of repeatedly swinging a golf club.

2. Getting your swing checked. A golf professional can analyze your swing to make sure it is safe for your back.
3. Getting back in the game gradually. If you haven't played golf all winter, slowly ease back into the game. Your body needs time to adapt to the demands of this sport.
4. Easing off the driver. Your driver and long irons create the most torque and are therefore the most likely to stress or strain your back. Try easing off 10% to 20%, and always swing smoothly and easily with these clubs.

Bowling

Two aspects of bowling are stressful to your back: (1) holding a ball at arm's length with the trunk flexed and (2) the twisting motion that occurs as the ball is released. Some tips to make this activity safer for your back include

1. Using the right size ball. Use a ball that you can release smoothly and easily. Avoid using a ball that is too heavy or doesn't fit your fingers well.
2. Having your form checked by a bowling professional. He or she can ensure that your technique is safe for your back.

▎ Healthy Eating

Studies have demonstrated that healthful eating is important to wound healing and general overall health. One of the best guides for sensible, healthy eating is the Mayo Clinic Healthy Weight Pyramid. The Mayo Clinic developed this pyramid to encourage long-term health, weight loss, and weight maintenance. The pyramid is scientifically based yet practical and easy to use. Some important aspects are

- A focus on low-energy dense foods (foods high in water and fiber). These foods help you feel full while eating fewer calories.
- An emphasis on choices within each food group that promote health.
- An unlimited amount (within your calorie allotment) of whole vegetables and fruit. Research has shown this is an effective practice in weight management.
- Putting physical activity in the center of the pyramid to encourage a central role for regular exercise and activity.

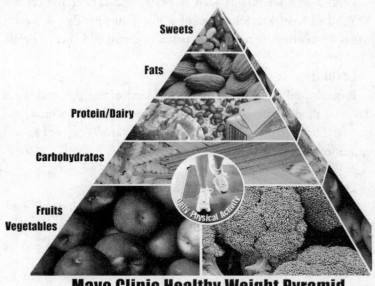

Mayo Clinic Healthy Weight Pyramid

From Mayo Clinic: Healthy Weight for Every Body © 2005. *Used with permission.*

Here is a level-by-level explanation of the Mayo Clinic Healthy Weight Pyramid. (For more information on the Mayo Clinic Healthy

Weight Pyramid, see the book *Mayo Clinic: Healthy Weight for Every Body*, which is available at bookstores and online retailers.)

Level 1

The base of the Mayo Clinic Healthy Weight Pyramid is an unlimited intake of vegetables and fruit with a minimum of 4 servings per day. Fresh vegetables and fruit are low-energy dense foods that occupy a large volume, take a relatively long time to eat, and are lower in calories than other foods.

Level 2

Level 2 is whole grains such as pasta, bread, rice, and cereals. You should have 4 to 8 servings of whole grains per day. A serving size is 70 calories: ½ cup of rice, pasta, or cereal or 1 slice of bread.

Level 3

Proteins and dairy occupy the third level of the pyramid. Each day, you should have 3 to 7 servings of beans, fish, lean meat, and low-fat dairy products. Serving size examples are ⅓ cup of beans, 3 ounces of meat or fish, or 1 cup of skim milk.

Level 4

Heart-healthy fats are at the fourth level. These include olive oil, nuts, such as almonds and walnuts, canola oil, and avocados. You should have 3 to 5 servings per day of heart-healthy fats. A serving size might be 1 teaspoon of olive oil or 1 tablespoon of nuts.

Level 5

Sweets such as candy, cookies, table sugar, and doughnuts comprise the top level. Use sparingly. Limit to 75 calories per day.

▋ Reaching and Maintaining Your Ideal Weight

Carrying extra weight is stressful for your back. Reaching and maintaining your ideal weight can help your back problem and improve your overall health.

What is a healthy weight for you?

A good way to find your healthy weight range is to check your body mass index (BMI). The BMI measures the relationship between your height and weight. To find your current BMI, use the chart. Find your height in the left-hand column. Move across to your weight. Your BMI is at the top of the column. For example, if you are 5 feet 5 inches tall (65 inches) and weigh 168 pounds, your BMI is 28. Shaded areas represent a healthy range.

BMI	19	20	21	22	23	24	25	26	27	28	29	30	31	32	33	34	35
Height (inches)	Body Weight (pounds)																
58	91	96	100	105	110	115	119	124	129	134	138	143	148	153	158	162	167
59	94	99	104	109	114	119	124	128	133	138	143	148	153	158	163	168	173
60	97	102	107	112	118	123	128	133	138	143	148	153	158	163	168	174	179
61	100	106	111	116	122	127	132	137	143	148	153	158	164	169	174	180	185
62	104	109	115	120	126	131	136	142	147	153	158	164	169	175	180	186	191
63	107	113	118	124	130	135	141	146	152	158	163	169	175	180	186	191	197
64	110	116	122	128	134	140	145	151	157	163	169	174	180	186	192	197	204
65	114	120	126	132	138	144	150	156	162	168	174	180	186	192	198	204	210
66	118	124	130	136	142	148	155	161	167	173	179	186	192	198	204	210	216
67	121	127	134	140	146	153	159	166	172	178	185	191	198	204	211	217	223
68	125	131	138	144	151	158	164	171	177	184	190	197	203	210	216	223	230

BMI	19	20	21	22	23	24	25	26	27	28	29	30	31	32	33	34	35
Height (inches)							**Body Weight (pounds)**										
69	128	135	142	149	155	162	169	176	182	189	196	203	209	216	223	230	236
70	132	139	146	153	160	167	174	181	188	195	202	209	216	222	229	236	243
71	136	143	150	157	165	172	179	186	193	200	208	215	222	229	236	243	250
72	140	147	154	162	169	177	184	191	199	206	213	221	228	235	242	250	258
73	144	151	159	166	174	182	189	197	204	212	219	227	235	242	250	257	265
74	148	155	163	171	179	186	194	202	210	218	225	233	241	249	256	264	272
75	152	160	168	176	184	192	200	208	216	224	232	240	248	256	264	272	279
76	156	164	172	180	189	197	205	213	221	230	238	246	254	263	271	279	287

SOURCE: National Heart, Lung, and Blood Institute, National Institutes of Health website.

A healthy BMI is between 19 and 25. If your BMI is less than 19, you are underweight. If it is greater than 25, you are overweight. To find your healthy weight range, find your height in the left-hand column. Now find the BMI number 19 along the top. Follow the row over from your height until you reach the column with the BMI of 19. This is your lowest healthy weight. To find your upper healthy weight, follow the row over from your height until you reach the column with the BMI of 25. For example, if you are 5 feet 7 inches tall (67 inches), your ideal weight should be between 121 and 153 pounds.

Losing Weight

Every year, billions of dollars are spent on losing weight. But every successful weight-loss program boils down to one central issue: *To lose weight, you have to eat less and/or exercise more.* To lose 1 pound in one week—a safe and sensible goal—you must burn 3,500 more calories than you eat (3,500 calories = 1 pound). That breaks down to about 500 calories per day. So you need to eat 500 calories less each day or burn 500 calories more by being active. Or you can balance it by eating a little less and exercising a little more. Here are five ways to easily cut 200 to 300 calories from your diet plus five ways to easily burn 200 to 300 extra calories in a day.

Five Ways to Cut 200 to 300 Calories	Calories Saved	Five Ways to Burn 200 to 300 Calories	Calories Burned
1. Eat one egg instead of two.	75	1. Walk for 30 minutes at 4 mph.	200
Eat an open-faced sandwich.	90		
Substitute 12 ounces of flavored water for soda.	<u>140</u>		
Total	**305**		
2. Eat an orange instead of drinking 8 ounces of orange juice.	50	2. Jog for 20 minutes at 5 mph.	200
Substitute 8 ounces of 1% milk for whole milk.	50		
Eat ½ cup of spaghetti instead of 1 cup.	<u>100</u>		
Total	**200**		
3. Substitute 3 ounces of roasted chicken breast without skin for 3 ounces of fried chicken with skin.	50	3. Perform 30 minutes of strength training.	200
Substitute 1 slice of light bread for regular.	50		
Have 1 cup of chicken noodle soup instead of beef chili with beans.	<u>100</u>		
Total	**200**		
4. Skip the 2-inch butterscotch brownie!	250	4. Play singles tennis for 30 minutes.	225

Five Ways to Cut 200 to 300 Calories	Calories Saved	Five Ways to Burn 200 to 300 Calories	Calories Burned
5. Have 1½ ounces of cheesecake instead of 3 ounces.	150	5. Do 1 hour of active housework.	250
Skip the cream in your coffee.	50		
Total	**200**		

Estimates of calories burned (expended) are based on a 150-pound person (e.g., a 100-pound person burns about 80 calories /mile; a 200-pound person will burn 130 calories/mile).

In general, to lose weight women should take in no more than 1,200 to 1,400 calories per day and men should take in no more than 1,400 to 1,600. *Be sure to check with your doctor before starting any weight-loss program.*

Some Helpful Hints for Losing Weight

1. Get support. Studies have shown that support can be helpful when trying to lose weight. Maybe you have a friend who would like to lose weight with you. Or join a weight-loss program with support groups such as Weight Watchers.

2. Increase your activity level throughout the day. Don't sit for more than thirty minutes. Take brief walking or stretching breaks throughout the day.

3. Drink more water. This makes you feel full, which lessens your cravings for food. Shoot for drinking eight 8-ounce glasses of water each day. You can count juice, herbal teas, other noncaffeinated fluids, and soup toward your eight glasses.

4. Increase your fiber intake by eating more vegetables, fruits, whole grains, and legumes. Strive to consume 25 to 30 grams of fiber per day. Fruit and vegetables are also important sources of vitamins and minerals.

5. Don't skip meals. Skipping meals makes you feel deprived, which increases your craving for food. Eating breakfast is especially important. Many experts consider skipping breakfast a big deterrent to losing weight. Instead of skipping meals, eat smaller portions. Between meals, eat small portions of healthful snacks.

6. Keep a food journal. Writing down what you eat has been repeatedly shown to help change eating habits and weight loss. Use a small notebook to write down everything you eat every day.

7. Shop smart. Shop mainly the store's perimeter for produce, low-fat dairy, and lean meats. Keep healthier foods in your cupboards and refrigerator. Stock up on low-calorie and healthy snacks as well as fruits and vegetables.

22

What Do I Do If My Surgery Doesn't Seem to Have Worked?

Occasionally, surgery for back problems doesn't work out the way it was intended. This has been called failed back surgery syndrome by some doctors and other people not familiar with the true issues. There are many reasons why surgery results are not always ideal. If you are a back patient whose surgery didn't work, the key issue is finding out why.

▌ Reasons That Back Surgery Can Fail

1. A back problem could be misdiagnosed or incompletely diagnosed. All good back treatment, especially surgery, depends on getting a good diagnosis. Surgery works best when the surgeon understands exactly what is wrong with your back and how to fix it. Unfortunately, sometimes the true source of a patient's pain is misdiagnosed. In this case, the surgeon thinks the patient's pain is coming from one problem when it is actually due to a different problem. For example, Dr. Winter recently saw a case at a conference in

which a patient had severe leg pain and an MRI that showed a disc bulge. The logical conclusion was that the disc bulge was pinching a nerve, thus causing the leg pain. The patient was scheduled for surgery to remove the disc bulge. At surgery, the nerve was swollen and irritated, but it was not compressed by the disc. Two days later, the patient exhibited shingles, a viral infection involving the nerves. This infection was causing the leg pain.

Another example of misdiagnosis is a patient with a herniated disc who is operated on at the wrong level. In this case, the operation should be performed again at the correct level, probably by a different surgeon.

If a back problem is incompletely diagnosed, surgery might help but may not completely fix the problem. For example, if a patient had surgery for a disc herniation with both back and leg pain and got good relief from the leg pain but continues to have major back pain, it is probably because the disc that was ruptured was also degenerated. The surgical answer is not another discectomy but rather to treat the degeneration with fusion surgery (or perhaps in the future with disc replacement surgery).

A similar situation can occur after decompression surgery for spinal stenosis. Nerve compression symptoms (pain, weakness, and/or numbness in the legs) may go away, yet increasing back pain occurs. This is caused by degeneration of the discs, not stenosis. If the pain is bad enough, the patient might need a second surgery—a fusion operation—to fix the degeneration. This is not a problem due to misdiagnosis, since the surgeon knew of the degeneration and hoped that the decompression would also help the back pain (which it often does). The surgeon wanted to spare the patient the additional trauma of a fusion operation.

2. The correct surgical procedure could be incompletely performed. Sometimes the surgeon will know exactly what is wrong and perform the correct surgery, but the patient will still have pain.

This may happen if the surgical procedure was not done thoroughly. For example, the patient might have decompression surgery for a pinched nerve (or nerves) in her back. If the decompression is not fully accomplished—that is, if whatever is pinching the nerve(s) is not cleaned out completely—the pinching may continue. In this case, a repeat laminectomy may be necessary after tests are done to confirm the problem.

3. A person may not respond well to surgery. Your body must respond to surgery in a predictable, healthy manner in order for it to be successful. This is particularly important for fusion surgery. The goal of any fusion surgery is to have two bones solidly fuse together. When a fusion fails and the two bones do not heal properly, it is called a pseudarthrosis (*pseudo* means "false" and *arthrosis* means "joint"). This is usually but not always a painful situation.

A fusion operation may fail to work or fuse for many reasons. Smoking, anemia (low blood count), diabetes, obesity, and inactivity have all been shown to hinder fusion healing.

If a patient has had a nonhealing fusion operation, the only way to eliminate the pain is to do further surgery to achieve a solid union of the two bones. It has been shown that going back into the old incision and just adding more bone graft often doesn't work. Better results are achieved by going in and doing more complex surgical work.

If a patient has had a typical lower back posterior fusion without instrumentation, the best results will probably come from adding an anterior interbody fusion plus redoing the posterior fusion and adding instrumentation. If a patient has had a typical lower back posterior fusion with instrumentation, the best results will probably come from adding an anterior interbody fusion, plus rechecking the posterior fusion, adding more bone graft, and tightening up the instrumentation or replacing it.

If a patient has had an anterior interbody fusion with a cage, the best results will probably come from redoing the anterior fusion with cage removal, adding bone graft anteriorly, then doing a posterior fusion with instrumentation. If a patient has had a thoracic scoliosis operation and a pseudarthrosis has been found, the best results will probably come from a posterior reoperation with more bone graft and replacement of the instrumentation. If a patient has had a posterior-only operation for a kyphosis problem and has a pseudarthrosis, then the best answer is adding an anterior fusion plus redoing the posterior operation.

4. A back problem may reoccur either in the same place or in a different place. Sometimes surgery successfully treats a patient's back problem, and a year or so later the pain comes back. If a patient had surgery for a disc herniation, this may mean the same disc has herniated again or a new herniation has occurred at another level. In either case, an MRI or CT myelogram will indicate the cause of the patient's pain, and a repeat surgery may be necessary.

Spinal stenosis is another problem that can come back in a different place. A patient may have had decompression surgery and done well for one to five years only to have the nerve compression symptoms come back. This is almost always due to a new compression occurring at a place in the spine that was just fine at the time of the earlier surgery.

Dr. Winter's secretary had a successful operation for spinal stenosis and degenerative disc disease (decompression and fusion). Five years later, her pain came back. Tests revealed that she had the same problem as before but in a different place. She had the same surgery done for the new problem and is doing just fine.

5. Surgery may cause a secondary problem. If screws and/or rods are used for a fusion operation, they can cause a localized irritation where the muscles rub over them. This is rare and can usually be solved be removing the screws and/or rods that are causing the problem.

▮ The Next Step

If you had spine surgery but continue to have a lot of pain, an evaluation by a good spine surgeon is your next step. This doctor will likely be able to tell you why you continue to hurt and whether further surgery might help. You should begin, of course, with your original surgeon, since the answer and treatment may be obvious. If, however, your original surgeon says that everything possible has been done and you'll just have to live with the pain, you must get another opinion from a good spine surgeon.

A good friend of mine (Dr. Winter's), a young resident physician, had two failed back surgeries (laminectomies). She was so miserable and needed so much pain medication that she could not perform her duties as a resident doctor. She was told by her neurosurgeon that everything possible had been done. She got a second opinion from a good spine surgeon, was properly diagnosed, and underwent appropriate fusion surgery. Now, five years later, she is completely pain-free and working full-time as a physician. She calls her decision to seek another opinion and have further surgery "the best decision of my life."

Don't adopt a nothing-more-can-be-done mindset. Seek another opinion! It is hard to see people chronically addicted to pain medications when their problem could be fixed.

There might not be a surgical answer to your problem. If that is true, your doctor can help you find the best solution for your situation. As we discussed in Chapter 18, our minds can powerfully affect how we heal and how much pain we have. Psychotherapy can help if the doctor determines that most of your pain is caused by errant mental or emotional processes.

You may have a back problem that cannot be repaired with further surgery. Psychotherapy can help you learn strategies for living with your pain. In addition, narcotic medication, an implanted spinal cord stimulator, or a morphine pump can be used to treat pain.

Finally, there may be a surgical answer to your problem, but you may decide you don't want surgery again. In this case, your doctor can help you make the best of your situation with pain medications, pain-control devices (such as a morphine pump), a referral to a chronic pain clinic, or a referral to psychotherapy.

23

Back Pain in Children and Adolescents

Back pain in children and adolescents is very different than in adults. Adults are subject to some types of back problems (disc herniation, degenerative facet joints, spinal stenosis, and degenerative spondylolisthesis) that children never have and adolescents have only rarely. Psychological and emotional issues, which can be a big component in adult back pain problems, are much rarer in children. Thus, if your child or adolescent complains of back pain, it is likely to be a real physical problem.

■ Spondylolysis and Spondylolisthesis

The most common cause of back pain in children is spondylolysis or spondylolisthesis. Spondylolyis is a defect in the posterior part of the vertebra; spondylolisthesis is a slipping forward of one vertebra on the other (see Fig. 8, p. 29). These conditions cause lower back pain and sometimes leg pain. The pain usually begins as a low-grade off-and-on pain and becomes more and more bothersome over time.

It is more common in athletes, especially in gymnasts and football linemen.

Spondylolysis can occur without spondylolisthesis—that is, the defect in the vertebrae is present without the slipping apart of the vertebrae. It is usually detected on routine X-rays, but sometimes special imaging such as a CT scan, MRI scan, or bone scan is required to detect it.

Many children with spondylolysis have no symptoms. In this case, no treatment is necessary and full activities are encouraged. Mild to moderate symptoms generally respond well to activity limitation and strengthening of the core muscles (particularly the abdominal, spinal, and gluteal muscles). Medications are used for very short durations to treat acute flare-ups.

Spondylolysis and spondylolisthesis may cause significant pain in children and adolescents and may keep them from the activities they enjoy. In this case, surgery—specifically spinal fusion—is the usual and customary treatment. The surgical technique depends on the child's age and the amount of deformity. The success rate is very high. If the child's symptoms include leg pain caused by pinched nerve roots, both nerve decompression and fusion are done.

In rare situations, the spondylolisthesis (the slipping of one vertebra on another) is significant, but the child has no symptoms. If the slipping is getting worse and worse, fusion surgery is done even if there is little or no pain. This is because there is the potential for the two vertebrae to completely fall apart, which is a serious problem that is very difficult to fix.

■ Scheuermann's Disease

Scheuermann's disease is a back condition characterized by an increase in thoracic kyphosis. It is the second most common cause of back pain in children. Scheuermann's disease becomes evident in adolescence and is not seen before age 10. The cause is unknown, but there is a strong genetic link (that is, it tends to run in families). It occurs equally in boys and girls.

Children with Scheuermann's disease are often brought to the doctor's office because the parents are concerned about the child's "bad posture." If indeed the problem is just bad posture, a physical examination and routine X-rays will be normal. However, if the physical examination and X-rays confirm the typical features of Scheuermann's disease, the child simply cannot stand straight or demonstrate good posture.

The most effective treatment for Scheuermann's disease is bracing. This treats the pain and/or the kyphosis. Treatment is carried out by spine surgeons who are trained in brace treatment or by pediatric orthopedists with good training in spine management. Surgery is seldom necessary if the brace is worn as prescribed. If the brace is not worn and the deformity gets worse, surgery is appropriate. In rare instances in which the deformity gets worse despite wearing the brace properly, surgery is also indicated. If the deformity is still flexible, surgery involves posterior instrumentation and fusion. If the deformity is rigid, then anterior release and fusion plus posterior instrumentation and fusion are done.

Physical therapy, medications, chiropractic, and other forms of nonsurgical treatment to correct posture and strengthen the back muscles have not proven effective for children with Scheuermann's disease.

▌ Premature Disc Degeneration

Disc degeneration is a common problem in adults, but it is rare in adolescents. Juvenile disc degeneration describes a condition in which the discs in an adolescent essentially age long before they normally should. The symptoms are back pain without leg pain.

In the past, children with back pain caused by juvenile disc degeneration were diagnosed as having psychosomatic problems (the cause of their pain was thought to be psychological, not physical). Now, with the development of MRI, doctors have determined that some adolescents do develop juvenile disc degeneration and that those with degeneration commonly have back pain.

▌Scoliosis

The most common type of scoliosis in adolescents is called idiopathic scoliosis. The word *idiopathic* means the cause is unknown. We do know that idiopathic scoliosis is strongly hereditary, usually running on the female side of the family. Most adolescents with this problem have no pain at all. A few, especially those with large curves, do have a mild aching pain in the curve area that is not bad enough to require medication. These are the curves that usually need surgery because of their size. Daily activities can be done without limitation. This is so typical that if a scoliosis patient comes in with a major pain problem, something else is usually causing the pain.

▌Spinal Cord Tumors

Spinal cord tumors are uncommon, but they are a very serious cause of back pain in children. They tend to occur in younger children rather than adolescents, but they can occur at any age. Because they involve the spinal cord, nerve-related symptoms such as leg pain, numbness, tingling, and weakness are common. Symptoms often begin, however, with only back pain. For this reason, it is extremely important for the doctor to do a thorough neurological examination if your child complains of back pain. Any complaint of night pain or difficulty sleeping should be taken seriously.

Routine X-rays seldom show a spinal cord tumor. MRI scans are ideal for making the diagnosis. The treatment is for a neurosurgeon to surgically remove the tumor. Some of these tumors are malignant (cancerous) and others are benign (noncancerous). Chemotherapy and radiation are seldom of any value.

■ Spinal Bone Tumors

Several different kinds of bone tumors are found in the spine of children and adolescents. Some are malignant and some are benign. One of the most common is a tumor called an osteoid osteoma. It is a small, completely benign tumor that can cause a great deal of pain. It is difficult to see on routine X-rays but "lights up" spectacularly with a bone scan. Treatment for this condition is surgical removal of the tumor by a spine surgeon.

A few years ago, one of the doctors at the Twin Cities Spine Center was called in to see a patient on the adolescent psychiatric unit of a local hospital. She was having behavioral problems and was constantly complaining of thoracic back pain. An osteoid osteoma was found. Once this was removed, her behavior improved dramatically.

Experiences like this one have led the Twin Cities Spine Center to develop a rule that no child or adolescent is diagnosed with psychosomatic back pain unless a thorough physical and neurological examination, routine X-rays, bone scan, and MRI all come back negative. A psychologist or psychiatrist must also concur with the diagnosis.

■ Other Back Problems in Children and Adolescents

Children and adolescents are active. They have falls and injuries that can cause back strains and sprains. These problems usually respond quickly to simple self-care. As with adults, major injuries can result in fractures or major ligament injuries, some of which may require surgical repair.

Disc herniations—so common in adults—are rare in children and adolescents. They can, however, occur and are best diagnosed by MRI scan. Surgical removal is necessary more often in children than in adults.

Psychosomatic causes of back pain are much less common in children than adults. They tend to occur in families that are either too chaotic or too rigid. If one or both parents have chronic back problems, a child is also at greater risk.

Gynecologic problems are often overlooked causes of back pain in adolescent girls. An evaluation by a female gynecologist is best.

Syringomyelia is a condition in which a cyst (fluid-filled cavity) develops in the spinal cord. This causes back pain and may cause symptoms of spinal cord malfunction such as weakness or numbness. It can also cause scoliosis. Syringomyelia is not a tumor, but it does require neurosurgical treatment.

Infections of the spine can occur in either young children or adolescents. Typically, bacteria that are in the bloodstream land in the spine. With the availability of antibiotics, these infections are unusual. Infections are most likely to be caused by common bacteria that are easily treated with antibiotics. A culture does not need to be obtained before treatment is started, contrary to the situation with adults. Children from underdeveloped countries may have tuberculosis, so they must have a culture done first. Surgery is rarely needed.

APPENDIX A

Resources

These resources will help you find the best practitioners and the most up-to-date information to support you in living well with back pain. We have provided categories for your convenience.

Advocacy/Making Decisions Books

How to Get Out of the Hospital Alive: A Guide to Patient Power
By Sheldon P. Blau and Elaine Shimberg
   This book, written by a doctor who had a "near-death" experience after heart surgery, is a no-nonsense primer that encourages hospital patients to be informed, vigilant, and protective of their health. It specifies actions that patients need to take before, during, and after a hospital visit to ensure safe treatment and a quick and uneventful recovery.

The Intelligent Patient's Guide to the Doctor–Patient Relationship:
Learning How to Talk So Your Doctor Will Listen
By Barbara Korsch and Caroline Harding
   This book's premise is that the relationship you form with your doctor directly relates to the quality of care you receive. The authors help you gain an equal footing with your doctors by assisting you in understanding the doctor–patient relationship and the unwritten rules that govern it.

Making Informed Medical Decisions: Where to Look and How to Use
What You Find
By Nancy Oster, Lucy Thomas, and Darol Joseff
   This book helps you identify and gain access to information resources regarding diagnosis and treatment options. It assumes knowledge of the Internet.

Take This Book to the Hospital with You

By Charles Inlander and Ed Weiner

This book empowers you to ask questions, to ask for information, and to exercise your right to say yes or no to a doctor's recommendations. Using the accurate metaphor of going to the hospital as going on a trip, it encourages you to learn how to avoid infection, to change your room (or doctor or nurse!), and to scrutinize your bill for errors.

Working with Your Doctor: Getting the Healthcare You Deserve

By Nancy Keene

This book gives you the facts you need to know in order to find the right doctor, communicate effectively, ask the right questions, and resolve problems when your care is compromised. It is an education in patient advocacy.

Back-Related Books

Back in Control: A Conventional and Complementary Prescription for Eliminating Back Pain

By David Borenstein

This book, written by a rheumatologist, emphasizes finding the correct diagnosis and being an educated consumer. Alternative therapies are discussed in detail.

Back Pain Remedies for Dummies

By Michael Sinel and William Deardorff

Dr. Sinel is a physical medicine and rehabilitation specialist who provides a comprehensive list of the things that can cause back pain, as well as the various tests and treatments. Dr. Hochschuler, an orthopedic spine surgeon, writes a chapter on surgery.

Back Sense: A Revolutionary Approach to Halting the Cycle of Chronic Back Pain

By Ronald D. Seigel, Michael H. Urdang, and Douglas R. Johnson

The premise of this book is that while most back pain may start with a physical injury or strain, the real cause of back pain is muscle tension and spasms due to stress and inactivity.

No More Aching Back
By Leon Root

This book, written by an orthopedic surgeon with a strong rehabilitation emphasis in his practice, gives an excellent overview of the problems that can cause back pain as well as the various tests and treatments available. A major emphasis is placed on a tailored physical therapy program.

Say Goodbye to Back Pain
By Emile Hiesiger and Marian Betancourt

This book, written by a neurologist and pain management expert, discusses spinal anatomy, spinal abnormalities that cause pain, and the various treatments available. Both surgical and nonsurgical treatments are discussed.

Treat Your Back without Surgery: The Best Non-Surgical Alternatives for Eliminating Back and Neck Pain
By Stephen Hochschuler and Bob Reznik

This is an interesting book—despite its title, 25% of the book has to do with spine surgery. This is not surprising since Dr. Hochschuler is an orthopedic spine surgeon. The main treatment emphasis is on physical therapy.

Treat Your Own Back
By Robin McKenzie

This book, written by a physical therapist, includes exercises focused on relieving pain. The primary emphasis is on extension exercises.

Your Aching Back: A Doctor's Guide to Relief
By Augustus White III

This book, written by a prominent orthopedic spine surgeon, gives a detailed picture of spine anatomy as well as the many different causes for back pain. Despite Dr. White's surgical profession, nonsurgical care is emphasized.

Back-Related Websites

www.spine-health.com

This website offers some good general information about what causes back pain, how it can be treated, and recent research about this topic. This site is sponsored by two of the largest sellers of spine implants: Medtronic and Johnson & Johnson.

www.back.com

This site is sponsored by Medtronic. It offers to help you find a doctor in your area, but it only lists surgeons who use Medtronic products.

www.aafp.org

This is the website of the American Academy of Family Practice, and it is one of the very best. It provides general facts about acute back pain, how to tell if your back problem requires emergency help, causes of back pain, and the customary tests and treatments for various back problems.

www.orthoinfo.aaos.org

This is the website of the American Academy of Orthopedic Surgeons, and it is a good one. This website lists various conditions and parts of the skeleton, so you need to go to the section on the spine and back pain. This site covers why low back pain is common, how it is diagnosed, when surgery may be helpful, and what exercises may be useful.

www.spine.org

The North American Spine Society website is the site for medical specialists who devote the majority of their practice to spine problems. Medical specialties include orthopedic surgery, neurosurgery, neurology, physical medicine and rehabilitation, and radiology.

www.srs.com

The website of the Scoliosis Research Society has excellent information on many kinds of back problems, not just scoliosis.

www.scoliosis-assoc.org

The Scoliosis Association, Inc., is the lay group for scoliosis and other spine problems, and it can be very helpful to those with questions and concerns.

www.neurosurgery.org

The website of the Neurosurgical Society is another source of reliable information on back problems.

The following are websites for back problem information sponsored by university medical centers:

www.healthcare.ucla.edu
   The website of the University of California at Los Angeles.

www.orthop.washington.edu
   The website of the orthopedic department at the University of Washington, Seattle.

www.lib.uiowa.edu
   The website of the University of Iowa.

www.mayoclinic.com
   Note: The Mayo Clinic is a private enterprise, not a university. The Mayo Clinic has its own medical school, and its website has excellent information on virtually every health topic including back problems.

General Health Information

Johns Hopkins Family Health Book
Edited by Michael J. Klag
   This is a massive (1,680 pages) home reference tool. It includes sections on body systems, health and nutrition, a color atlas of anatomy disorders and diseases, first aid, medications, lab tests, and so forth.

   The following resources are listed for those who may have specific questions, concerns, or complaints:

Americans with Disabilities Act
Technical Assistance Center
800-514-0301 (voice) or 800-514-0383 (TTY/TDD)

Centers for Medicare & Medicaid Service
7500 Security Blvd.
Baltimore, MD 21244-1850
877-267-2323
www.cms.hhs.gov/

Medicare Coordination of Benefits
P.O. Box 5041
New York, NY 10274-5041
800-999-1118 (voice) or 800-318-8782 (TTY/TDD)
www.cms.hhs.gov/medicare/cob

National Association of Insurance Commissioners
Executive Headquarters
2301 McGee St.
Suite 800
Kansas City, MO 64108-2662
816-842-3600
www.naic.org

U.S. Department of Labor
Employee Benefits Security Administration
Frances Perkins Building
200 Constitution Ave., NW
Washington, DC 20210
866-444-3272 (voice) or 877-889-5627 (TTY/TDD)
www.dol.gov/ebsa/

Finding Doctors/Verifying Credentials

American Board of Medical Specialties
1007 Church St. #404
Evanston, IL 60201
800-733-2267
www.abms.org.htm
    You can find out at this source whether a physician is board certified and
in what specialty.

American Medical Association
515 N. State St.
Chicago, IL 60610
312-464-5000

www.ama-assn.org/aps/amahg.htm
Here you can find out if a doctor is a member of the AMA (many are not) and what specialty the doctor practices.

American Board of Family Practice
2228 Young Dr.
Lexington, KY 40505
859-269-5626
www.aafp.org
Here you can find out if a family practice doctor is board certified.

American Board of Neurological Surgery
6550 Fannin St.
Suite 2139
Houston, TX 77030-2701
713-441-6015
www.abns.org
Here you can find out if a neurosurgeon is board certified.

American Board of Orthopaedic Surgery
400 Silver Cedar Court
Chapel Hill, NC 27514
919-929-7103
www.abos.org
Here you can find out if an orthopedic surgeon is board certified.

American Board of Physical Medicine and Rehabilitation
3015 Allegro Park Lane SW
Rochester, MN 55902
507-282-1776
www.abpmr.org
Here you can find out if a physiatrist is board certified.

The following websites provide information about these specialties:

Neurosurgery
www.aans.org

Orthopedic Surgery
www.orthoinfo.aaos.org

Physical Medicine and Rehabilitation
www.apmr.org

Back Support Groups

By and large, the websites for these groups provide resources for patients:

National Scoliosis Foundation
www.scoliosis.org/forum/php

Scoliosis Association, Inc.
www.scoliosis-assoc.org

Spondlyitis Association of America
www.spondylitis.org

Back Organizations

These groups are dedicated to research and clinical study, so their websites are primarily resources for physicians and secondarily for interested laypersons.

International Society for the Study of the Lumbar Spine
www.issls.org

North American Spine Society
www.spine.org

Scoliosis Research Society
www.srs.org

Mind/Back Connection Books

The Complete Idiot's Guide to Managing Stress
By Jeff Davidson

Stress has been shown to be a leading factor behind all sorts of mental and physical health problems and illnesses. This book offers an array of options to manage your stress, including organizing your day, on-the-spot exercises to relieve pressure, what to do when you're really stressed out, and more.

Full Catastrophe Living: Using the Wisdom of Your Body and Mind to Face Stress, Pain and Illness
By Jon Kabat-Zinn

This book is the basis of the MBSR (mindfulness-based stress reduction) course that was developed at the University of Massachusetts Medical School. It details the program, which uses mindfulness meditation to teach those with chronic illness and pain how to pay attention to the pain, live in the awareness of the moment, and spend time being rather than doing.

Healing Back Pain: The Mind–Body Connection
By John Sarno

Dr. Sarno's book promotes the theory that repressed anxiety causes emotional tension, which in turn causes muscular tension, resulting in back pain. The primary treatment is thus psychological.

Healing Back Pain Naturally: The Mind–Body Program Proven to Work
By Art Brownstein

This book is similar to Dr. Sarno's, but it includes diet and physical therapy in addition to mental empowerment for the treatment of back pain. Dr. Brownstein is very negative about surgery except for certain emergency problems, despite his having a successful herniated disc removal.

Learned Optimism: How to Change Your Mind and Your Life
By Martin Seligman

Seligman, a former president of the American Psychological Association, presents cognitive techniques to help people undo lifelong habits of pessimism and related depression.

The Relaxation Response

By Herbert Benson

This was a groundbreaking book in 1975, showing that meditation and relaxation have measurable effects on blood pressure and heart rate.

The Relaxation and Stress Reduction Workbook, 5th ed.

By Martha Davis, Elizabeth Robbins Eshelman, and Matthew McKay

This comprehensive (280 pages) resource includes information and exercises focused on breathing, relaxation, meditation, thought-stopping, body awareness, triggers to diffuse conflict, goal setting, time management, and assertiveness. It's a well-rounded resource.

Stress Management for Dummies

By Allen Elkin

After helping to determine your stress level, this book offers ways to eliminate the sources of stress.

Walking Books

ACSM's Guidelines for Exercise Testing and Prescription, 6th ed.

By the American College of Sports Medicine

This book is the in-depth, authoritative guide to scientifically based exercise testing and prescriptions. It is written for professionals in the field and interested laypersons.

Fitness Walking

By Therese Iknoian

This book contains everything you need to know to start a walking program, complete with color-coded program guides. It is an excellent resource for beginners.

Prevention's Complete Book of Walking

By Maggie Spilner

This book provides all the tools and techniques to help the walker get the most from his or her walking routine.

ShapeWalking: Six Easy Steps to Your Best Body
By Marilyn L. Bach and Lorie Schleck
This excellent resource coaches those interested in a low-cost fitness program by combining fitness walking, strength training, and spot shaping for specific areas of the body.

Walking: A Complete Guide to the Complete Exercise
By Casey Meyers
From stroll to brisk walk to aerobic walk to race walking, this book (now considered a classic) explains the best techniques for each speed and how to make progress from the first level to the last.

Walking Websites

Leslie Sansom's video Walk the Walk: Cardio
www.collagevideo.com
This is a low-impact aerobic video at the beginning/intermediate level for those interested in walking for recovery.

"Physical Activity and Health: A Report of the Surgeon General,"
Online/Centers for Disease Control Website
www.cdc.gov/nccdphp/sgr/ataglan.htm
This oft-quoted government reference emphasizes the importance of thirty minutes of moderate activity most days for everyone. It includes information on strength training for older adults and making activity a regular part of life.

Physical Therapy Books

8 Minutes in the Morning
By Jorge Cruise
The emphasis here is on strength training, with simple daily routines, advice on diet, and lots of encouragement.

The Back Pain Book: A Self-Help Guide for Daily Relief of Neck and Back Pain
By Mike Hage
This book emphasizes posture and body movement during everyday activities. Specific diagnoses are not discussed.

Staying Strong: A Senior's Guide to a More Active and Independent Life
By Lorie Schleck

Focusing on everyday activities, this book presents easy, progressive programs for strength training, balance, and flexibility.

Physical Therapy Website

Collage Video
www.collagevideo.com

In addition to a wide selection of videos and DVDs for aerobics, stretching, and toning, this site offers specialty selections appropriate for those with mobility issues and chronic health conditions. Resources for guided sitting exercises are available.

Yoga/Pilates Books

30 Essential Yoga Poses for Beginning Students and Their Teachers
By Judith Lasater

This book is highlighted for its clarity and detail in teaching the fundamental physical poses. It includes sequences for daily practice and a "theme" series for those wishing to focus on the lower back, hips, and so forth, or on a specific practice for energy or relaxation.

The Complete Guide to Joseph H. Pilates' Techniques of Physical Conditioning
By Allan Menezes

Pilates exercises offer a valuable fitness system, and this book includes three levels of workouts to increase strength and flexibility, reduce stress, and increase energy. This new edition includes many back-related exercises.

The Healing Path of Yoga
By Nischala Joy Devi

The author created the yoga component of Dr. Dean Ornish's original lifestyle program to reverse heart disease. The book's chair yoga exercises help promote spine flexibility and strength in a safe and gentle way.

The Woman's Book of Yoga & Health
By Linda Sparrowe
   In addition to yoga sequences by Patricia Walden, one of the premier Iyengar-style yoga teachers in the United States, the chapter on "Caring for Your Back" includes valuable information on how yoga can address kyphosis, scoliosis, and general back pain.

Yoga/Pilates Websites

Hugger Mugger Yoga Products
www.huggermugger.com
800-473-4888
   This company is good for yoga, Pilates, and meditation supplies.

Living Arts
www.Gaiam.com
800-254-8464
   This company is good for yoga, Pilates, and meditation supplies.

Yoga Fit
www.yogafit.com/teachers
   This site will help you find a qualified yoga teacher.

Yoga Journal
www.yogajournal.com
   Like the magazine, this is a comprehensive resource for finding supplies, a teacher, events, retreats, and solid advice.

Yoga/Pilates Videos and DVDs

AM and PM Yoga for Beginners
   With Rodney Yee and Patricia Walden

Pilates Beginning Mat Workout
   With Ana Caban

Yoga Journal's Practice Series
(various topics, led by Patricia Walden and Rodney Yee)
These videos and DVDs are recommended for home practice.

Healthy Nutrition and Weight-Control Books

2005 Mayo Clinic Healthy Weight for Everybody
Edited by Donald D. Hensrud
This attractive book lays out a complete, healthy lifestyle approach. The Healthy Weight Program includes twelve weeks of menus, recipes, and weight-loss strategies. Especially helpful is the "Action Guide to Weight-Loss Barriers," which will help consumers get past common mental/emotional obstacles. Its pyramid is presented in Chapter 21 of this book.

The Aerobics Program for Total Well-Being: Exercise, Diet,
Emotional Balance
By Kenneth H. Cooper
First published in 1982, this book provides simple, proven guidelines to support a balanced, complete fitness program. It demonstrates the correlation between various levels of physical activity and measurable health and risk-reduction benefits.

Carbohydrate Fat and Calorie Guide
By Jane Stephenson and Bridget Wagener
This handy pocket guide includes counts for all food groups, condiments, fast food, and generic restaurant food. It also lists vegetarian food and charts for estimating daily nutrient goals as well as estimates for calories burned while engaged in various activities. Most notable is that it provides detailed information on carbohydrates, fats, protein, fiber, and calories.

Eat, Drink and Be Healthy: The Harvard Medical School Guide to
Healthy Eating
By Walter C. Willette
This book emphasizes the key components for good health. The author was an early proponent of consuming healthy fats.

Effective Strength Training
By Douglas Brooks
This book is included because strength training is an important if not essential component of healthy weight maintenance.

Fitness and Health, 5th ed.
By Brian J. Sharkey
This book by a fitness authority is geared more for the professional and the performance athlete. Yet it presents an overall case for, and a program designed around, increasing activity and muscular fitness.

The Step Diet Book: Count Steps, Not Calories to Lose Weight and Keep It Off Forever
By James O. Hill
Walking has been shown to be one of the most effective, accessible, and high-compliance exercises to increase weight loss and improve health. Instead of counting calories, this guide helps change your mindset to counting steps, with long-lasting results.

Volumetrics: Feel Full on Fewer Calories
By Barbara Rolls and Robert A. Barnett
This book is based on the "science of satiety," or how low-density (low calories and high volume) foods make you feel satisfied. It helps you to lose weight without feeling hungry or deprived.

Healthy Nutrition and Weight-Control Websites

BMI Calculator
www.nhlbisupport.com/bmi/bmicalc.htm
This National Institutes of Health site uses the relationship of height and weight to calculate the body mass index, a measure of body fat that applies to adults.

Walk Off Weight (WOW) Plan from Prevention Magazine
http://prevention.genesant.com/
This program is a paid subscription. Before subscribing, there is a free ten-day trial that includes walking plans plus guidance on muscle toning and diets.

Diet Plans and Weight-Loss Programs
www.ediets.com
  By paid subscription, this site offers twenty-two personalized plans, with support and articles.

Health, Fitness, and Exercise Products
www.bodytrends.com

Health Tools from Acknowledged Experts
www.mayoclinic.com

Calorie Calculator
www.mayoclinic.com/health/calorie-calculator/NU00598#resulttext
  This tool helps you estimate your approximate daily calorie expenditure using height, weight, age, and activity level.

10,000 Steps Program by Shape Up America!
www.shapeup.org/10000steps.html
  This program by a nonprofit organization puts the emphasis on adding 2,000 steps to your baseline to maintain a healthy weight.

Walking and Weight Control
www.walking.about.com
  This site includes information on walking for fitness, exercise, weight loss, and competitive race walking. There are articles and a chat room.

Weight Loss Program
www.WeightWatchers.com
  This site includes information on local meetings plus online e-tools.

"Dietary Guidelines for Americans 2005," Online brochure/U.S.
Department of Agriculture and U.S. Department of Health and Human
Services Website
www.healthierus.gov/dietaryguidelines.htm.
  This report presents a format that can be individualized to your needs and stresses the necessity of physical activity.

USDA Food Pyramid
www.mypyramid.gov

This government site presents a format for healthy eating as well as recommendations for activity most days of the week.

Surgery Books

Surgery: A Patient's Guide from Diagnosis to Recovery
By Claire Mailhot, Melinda Brubaker, and Linda Garratt Slezak

The authors are nurses, educators, and administrators who provide surgical services. This book provides step-by-step information to help you and your family ensure the best outcome following surgery.

Understanding Your Spine Surgery, 2nd ed.
By Allina Health System Press
Inquiries to:
Allina Health System Press
710 E. 24th St.
Suite 400
Minneapolis, MN 55404
800-605-3744

This manual is a comprehensive guide that includes chapters on preparation for surgery as well as the hospital stay, discharge, and recovery. Detailed chapters on how to perform daily tasks and how to move most efficiently after surgery are particularly helpful.

Surgery Website

"Pre-surgery and Post-surgery Instructions," Online/University of Pittsburgh Medical Center Website
http://patienteducation.upmc.com/Pdf/Presurgery.pdf

These instructions are the basics that everyone having surgery needs to know. They are clearly organized and presented.

Medical Research Website

National Institutes of Health
www.ncbi.nlm.nih.gov/entrez/query

PubMed is the Internet site of the National Institutes of Health (NIH), our government agency responsible for health issues. PubMed contains scientific medical articles. Doctors use this site to find the latest published research articles on any given health topic. Although this is an excellent resource for health professionals, the medical and scientific articles would be very difficult for the average person to read and understand. There are about a thousand scientific articles published each year related to back pain. Access this site if you are particularly motivated to find the latest information and to wade through the medical and scientific jargon of the articles.

Advance Medical Directives Websites

National Hospice and Palliative Care Organization
www.caringinfo.org
800-658-8898
This site provides access to free, downloadable state-specific advance directive documents and instructions.

Five Wishes Health Care Directive
www.agingwithdignity.org/5wishes.html
888-5wishes (594-7437)
This form, in plain English and Spanish, meets legal requirements in thrity-seven states and the District of Columbia. In the other thirteen states, it can still be useful as an attachment to the state's required forms.

APPENDIX B

Glossary

Acupuncture The ancient Chinese technique of placing fine needles along certain "pathways" on the body (see Chapter 3).

Aerobic Exercise Exercise that gets the heart pumping and increases oxygen uptake. Includes activities such as walking, swimming, biking, and running. Helps make the heart and circulatory system healthier.

Allograft A bone graft obtained from another person or cadaver.

Analgesia A medication to reduce pain.

Ankylosing Spondylitis An inflammatory arthritis that usually involves the spine and sacroiliac joints. It frequently leads to spontaneous fusion.

Annulus (Annulus Fibrosis) The tough outer layer of fibrous tissue surrounding the disc.

Arachnoditis Irritation or inflammation of the nerve roots of the cauda equina leading to binding of the roots to one another.

Arthritis Inflammation of a joint, which can be degenerative, rheumatological, or infectious.

Arthrodesis *See* **Fusion**.

Artificial Disc Replaces a painful, degenerated disc. Several different types are being developed (see Chapter 4).

Autogenous Bone Graft A bone graft that comes from you, not another person or a cadaver.

Automatic Thoughts Positive or negative thoughts occurring outside one's awareness—in the unconscious—that influence beliefs, feelings, behavior, and the experience of pain.

Back Care Education Learning to sit, stand, lift, bend, and move in a way that causes the least stress to the back.

Back Care Pyramid A logical, evidence-based guide through back care options, starting with the easiest and least expensive treatments. For those who need it, each ascending level directs them to the right doctor and explains what to expect from each specialist on the pyramid.

Bedside Manner A doctor's interpersonal skill and ability to communicate.

Biofeedback Training Involves placing electrodes on the skin to monitor physical processes (such as heart rate or muscle tension). A monitor provides the person with direct feedback about these processes in order to learn how to control them.

BMI (Body Mass Index) Measures the relationship between height and weight in order to assess whether a person is at a healthy weight.

BMP (Bone Morphogenetic Protein) Naturally occurring substance in the body that is created when a person has a fracture that needs healing. Scientists have learned how to create it artificially. It is used to augment spine fusions (see Chapter 4).

Body Mechanics Moving and using the body, especially the back, in the safest manner.

Bone Scan A test in which a radioactive substance is injected into a vein. This substance tends to go to where there is inflammation and is read on a special counter.

Cage A metallic or plastic device that is filled with bone graft or bone morphogenetic protein and inserted between two vertebrae after removal of the disc (see Chapter 4).

Cauda Equina "Horse's tail." The bundle of nerves inside the dural sac in the lumbar spine below the end of the spinal cord.

Chemonucleolysis A common treatment before the 1990s for painful discs. An enzyme was injected into the disc, which dissolved the center. It is no longer used.

Coccyx The tip end of the sacrum—the tailbone.

Coordination of Benefits The section of a health insurance contract that explains how a medical treatment will be paid for if more than one insurer offers coverage for the treatment.

Copayments *See* **Out-of-Pocket Expenses.**

CT (CAT) Scan (Computed Axial Tomography) A special X-ray test that gives three-dimensional detail of bone structures.

CT Myelogram A test in which a myelogram is done followed by a CT scan. This provides information not obtainable by either CT alone or myelogram alone.

Decompression Surgical removal of whatever might be pressing on the spinal cord or nerves (see Chapter 4).

Decompressive Laminectomy An operation to remove a portion of the bone overlaying a compressed nerve.

Deductibles *See* **Out-of-Pocket Expenses.**

Deconditioning A reduction of activities in an effort to alleviate pain or for other reasons. Results in decrease in size, strength, and flexibility of muscles, as well as diminishment of cardiovascular and muscular endurance, often making a condition worse.

Degenerative Disc Disease A process by which the normally bouncy and rubbery disc loses its flexibility due to biochemical changes. It may or may not be painful.

Degenerative Spondylolisthesis The slipping forward of one vertebra on another due to degenerative changes in the disc and facet joints. This is most commonly seen at L4–L5.

Desk Review *See* **Formal Appeal.**

Discectomy The surgical removal of all or part of an intervertebral disc.

Discitis Infection in the disc space.

Discography A test in which a needle is inserted into the disc and a dye is injected. Both the pain response and the X-ray appearance of the disc are evaluated.

Dura (dural sac) The fibrous tube that contains the spinal cord, cauda equina, and spinal fluid.

Duration How long the individual engages in an activity.

Elective Treatments Medications, surgeries, or other procedures for a specific condition that a health insurer considers optional.

EMG (Electromyogram) A test involving the placement of fine needles into various muscles and reading the electrical impules given off by the muscles.

Empowerment The belief that an individual has the ability and resources to bring about the best possible outcome under any circumstance. The opposite of passivity.

Epidural Abscess A collection of pus in the space between the dural sac and the walls of the spinal canal.

Epidural Space The space between the dural sac and the walls of the spinal canal (see Chapter 2).

Ergonomics The study of how the body interacts with its environment at work, during sports, and in other settings. Also called human engineering. Concerned with the characteristics of people that need to be considered in designing and arranging things so that people and things will interact most effectively and safely.

Evidence-Based Medicine Medicine that has been scientifically proven to be more effective than either the body's own ability to heal itself or the healing effects of a placebo.

Exclusions or Limitations on Coverage Treatments that are not covered or are limited under a particular health insurance policy.

Experimental Treatments The newest medications, surgeries, and other procedures for a specific condition. They may not be covered by health insurance.

Extension Backward bending of the spine.

External Review Forty-one states and the District of Columbia have laws that provide for external reviews (sometimes called level 2 reviews) to resolve disputes between consumers and their health plans. This level of review involves people who are *not* representatives of a person's plan.

External Review Organization (ERO) Some states contract with private firms called EROs to handle the external review process and interface with the consumer.

Facetectomy The surgical removal of the facet joint.

Facet Joint The small joints in the back of the spine where two vertebrae contact each other (see Chapter 2).

Facet Rhizotomy The surgical procedure wherein the small nerves around the facet joint are destroyed, usually by radiofrequency.

Femoral Ring A piece of allograft bone obtained from the femur (thigh) bone.

Fibromyalgia The name given to a condition with fatigue and multiple areas of tenderness. *Fibro* means "fibrous tissue" and *algia* means "pain."

First Report of Injury Form A form that must be filed to begin authorizations for treatment due to on-the-job injuries.

Flexion Forward bending of the spine.

Foraminal Stenosis Narrowing of the foramen, the "hole" where the nerve passes out of the spine (see Chapter 2).

Formal Appeal A detailed grievance process with an insurance company, usually in writing.

Fortitude The ability and the willingness to cope with whatever circumstances come up. Accepting and being willing to do what needs to be done.

Frequency How often an individual engages in an activity.

Fusion Refers to both the surgical procedure of "welding" a joint together and the end result, a solid fusion (synonymous with arthrodesis).

General Orthopedic Surgeon An orthopedic surgeon or orthopedist specializes in the care of musculoskeletal system disorders (bones, joints, muscles, tendons, and ligaments). A general orthopedist will see a broad variety of orthopedic patients such as those with ankle sprains, knee strains, or back pain. An orthopedist may prescribe medications, recommend a nonsurgical treatment, or refer you to a spine specialist or spine surgeon.

General Rehabilitation Medical Doctor *See* **Physiatrist.**

Good Standing Posture Places the body in balanced upright alignment in which there is minimal muscle effort and the body is comfortable, not strained.

Guided Imagery Involves allowing another person, or audiotape, to guide someone into a state of relaxation. Can involve progressive muscle relaxation techniques.

Health Care Directive Document that gives legally binding guidance to family members and the health care team about wishes for medical care in the event that a patient can't communicate. Also known as an advance directive.

Health Insurance Premiums *See* **Out-of-Pocket Expenses.**

Herniated Disc A condition in which the inner core of the disc extrudes back into the spinal canal. This puts direct pressure on the nerve, which can cause pain to radiate all the way down the individual's leg to the foot.

Hyperkyphosis An amount of kyphosis that is beyond normal.

Hyperlordotic An amount of lordosis that is beyond normal.

Hypnosis Performed by a trained medical professional, it involves creating a state of focused concentration in order to relax the mind and the body.

IDET (Intervertebral Disc Electrothermography) A technique in which a special needle is placed into a disc and tissues are heated electrically (see Chapter 3).

Implant A device that a surgeon places inside a patient during surgery. An artificial disc is an implant. A pedicle screw rod construct is an implant. An intervertebral cage is an implant.

Indemnity Policy A health insurance plan that (1) imposes few restrictions on which health care providers someone sees and (2) picks up the costs for covered treatments after the insured pays a certain amount out-of-pocket, usually 20% of the treatment fee.

Informal Appeal An appeal for denial of payment of benefits, usually through a phone call to the insurance company's customer service department.

Intensity How much effort the individual puts into an activity, generally considered in terms of speed or resistance.

Internal Review The process that a health insurer uses to resolve disputes about the benefits it is legally obligated to provide. Internal reviews often consist of an *informal* appeal handled mainly via phone contacts with health plan members and a *formal* appeal that involves a detailed review of documents relating to a dispute.

Intramuscular Injections of pain medications typically into a muscle.

Intrathecal Fluid-filled space between the thin layers of tissue that cover the brain and spinal cord. Drugs can be injected into the fluid or a sample of the fluid can be removed for testing.

Intravenous Medications administered through a vein, usually in the arm.

Isthmic Spondylolisthesis The slipping forward of one vertebra on another due to a bone defect in the posterior arch, a spondylolysis, usually L5 on S1.

Joint Mobilization A manual technique directed at joints to restore function, decrease pain, and restore mobility.

Kyphoplasty The technique of placing a large needle into a vertebral body that has a compression fracture. A balloon is then passed down the needle into the vertebral body, inflated to restore height to the fractured bone, and then bone cement or another substance is inserted to maintain the restored height (see Chapter 4).

Kyphosis A posterior (backward) curvature in the spine. The thoracic spine is normally kyphotic.

Lamina The portion of a vertebra arching over the spinal canal (see Chapter 2).

Laminectomy The surgical removal of a vertebral lamina.

Laminotomy The surgical removal of a portion of the lamina, usually associated with a herniated disc fragment removal.

Laparoscopic Surgery A thin tube is inserted through a small incision in the skin, and tissue or organs are removed through it. It is generally a low-level invasive kind of surgery that produces less scarring and has a quicker recovery time than conventional surgery.

Level One Appeal *See* **Formal Appeal.**

Level Two Review *See* **External Review.**

Ligamentum Flavum Yellow ligament. This is a strong ligament in the back of the spine connecting one lamina to another.

Lordosis An anterior (forward) curvature of the spine. The cervical and lumbar spines are normally lordotic.

Managed Care Policy A health insurance plan that (1) charges a monthly premium to cover most or all medical care and (2) places restrictions on which health care providers can be seen and what treatments they can provide.

Mechanical Traction This method uses a mechanical device to create traction, or separation, of the vertebrae in the spine. Though popular a decade or so ago, mechanical traction is used infrequently now.

Medial Facetectomy The surgical procedure of a portion of a facet joint in order to decompress a nerve root.

Medicaid A form of health insurance created by federal law and designed to provide medical benefits for people with a low income. States have wide latitude to determine who is eligible for Medicaid and what benefits the program will offer.

Medical Specialist Any medical physician except a family practitioner or a general practitioner.

Medicare A form of health insurance created by federal law and designed for people over age 65. Medicare Part A provides coverage for hospital-based medical treatments. Additional Medicare coverages are available for a monthly premium.

Meditation Involves the intentional self-regulation of a person's attention. This is done by holding the focus of a person's attention on, for example, a word, a sound, the breath, a mantra, or a religious symbol.

Mental Imagery/Visualization A relaxation technique using a person's own mental images and sensory memories, which creates a calm and peaceful internal state.

Mindset The mental and emotional approach brought to bear on any situation or problem.

Mobility Exercises Exercises aimed at increasing and/or improving a person's ability to move in daily life.

MRI (Magnetic Resonance Imaging) A test done in a radiology department or radiology facility that does not involve the use of X-rays.

Multiple Myeloma A cancer of the bone marrow that often involves the spine.

Muscle Energy Techniques (MET) A manual technique used to restore normal position and motion to the lumbar segments. A physical therapist applies resistance to the contraction of specific muscles while the patient is prepositioned to facilitate the correct movement of segments or joints.

Myelogram A radiological test in which a needle is placed into the spinal fluid area, a dye is injected, and X-rays are taken.

Myofascial Release/Massage Involves vigorous massaging of tight soft tissue to release spasms, increase circulation, and improve extensibility (the ability of a tissue to move easily).

Narcotic A medication that tends to produce a sleepy feeling. Narcotics are strong pain medications, but they are also highly addictive.

Negative Thoughts Thoughts that negatively distort reality, create heavy emotions (such as anxiety, depression, and fear), and increase pain.

Nerve Conduction Studies When stimulated by a low dose of electricity, these studies test the response of the nerves in the legs or arms. The results help determine if a nerve is damaged or compromised.

Nerve Root The portion of a nerve as it comes out of the spinal cord and passes out the foramen.

Network An approved list of health care providers for a managed care plan. The plan may offer reduced coverage or no coverage at all for services from providers not on the list.

Neurological Deficit A loss of normal neurological function such as muscle strength, sensation, or reflexes. This loss can range from very mild (a little numbness) to very severe (complete paralysis).

Neurologist Spine Specialist Specializes in the diagnosis and nonsurgical treatment of brain and nervous system disorders. Often serves as a consultant, especially in distinguishing a primary neurological problem from a musculoskeletal one.

Nucleotomy The technique of inserting something into the disc space with the concept of dissolving or removing the disc contents.

Nucleus (Nucleus Pulposis) The soft, central part of the disc.

Nurse Practitioner Registered nurse with advanced training in a specialty such as adult or geriatric care. An NP performs many of the services done by doctors, often with an emphasis on nurturing and education, and always under the supervision of a doctor.

Occupational Therapist Helps to improve a person's ability to perform daily activities safely and efficiently and recommends home and job adaptations.

Optimism The potent combination of positive outlook and hope. The belief that even if things are difficult now, they can get better in the future.

Oral Medication Medication taken by mouth.

Orthopedic Spine Specialist An orthopedist specializing in back problems who knows the latest in diagnosis and treatment.

Orthopedic Spine Surgeon Focuses practice on the surgical care of back problems. Tends to perform surgery for herniated discs, scoliosis and kyphosis, disc degeneration (spinal fusion), and spinal stenosis (decompression).

Osteoid Osteoma A very painful but benign (noncancerous) bone tumor sometimes seen in the spine.

Osteomyelitis Infection in a bone. This can happen in the vertebral bodies in the spine.

Osteoporosis A condition in which the bones *(osteo)* do not have the normal density and strength *(porosis)*.

Out-of-Pocket Expenses Any costs for health care that must be paid by the insured before health insurance coverage applies. Examples of out-of-pocket expenses are health insurance premiums, deductibles, payments for out-of-network providers, and copayments or coinsurance.

Pacing Taking regular breaks so that the spine is not in the same position for too long.

Pars Interarticularis "The part between the articulations." The area of the posterior vertebral arch where a spondylolysis often occurs, the "pars defect."

Payments for Out-of-Network Providers *See* **Out-of-Pocket Expenses.**

PCA Pump Patient-controlled analgesia pump. It allows the patient to adjust the dose of pain medication directly into the bloodstream by pushing a hand-held button.

Pedicle A part of each vertebra; one on each side connecting the vertebral body to the lamina.

Pedicle Screw A bone screw placed down the pedicle.

Pedometer A small battery-run device that senses motion. It attaches to the waistband and counts the number of steps a person takes, walking and moving, throughout the day.

Peritoneum A membrane in the abdomen that covers the internal organs and creates a potential cavity in which fluids can collect.

Physiatrist Practices a medical specialty called physical medicine and rehabilitation (PM&R), utilizing a wide variety of conservative treatments for musculoskeletal disorders, but does not perform surgery. Physiatrists typically treat the whole person, addressing physical, mental, and emotional issues.

Physiatrist Spine Specialist A physiatrist who is a spine specialist (with more than 90% of practice focused on spine patients) and who offers more specialized diagnostic and treatment knowledge and experience.

Physical Medicine and Rehabilitation (PM&R) *See* **Physiatrist.**

Physical Therapist PTs provide services that help restore function, improve mobility, relieve pain, and prevent or limit permanent physical disabilities of patients suffering from injuries or disease. They restore, maintain, and promote overall fitness and health.

Physician Extender Cares for patients under the supervision of a physician. Nurse practitioners (NPs) and physician's assistants (PAs) are examples of physician extenders. They may also serve as primary care practitioners.

Physician's Assistant A college graduate who has completed an accredited physician's assistant program that is approximately twenty-six months in length. A physician's assistant becomes licensed by passing a national certification exam. A PA is a representative of the physician, treating patients in a manner developed and directed by the supervising physician.

Pilates A special type of exercise program that concentrates on the "core" muscles (trunk and abdominal). The name comes from its inventor (see Chapter 3).

Placebo A pill or procedure that is known to have no active action against whatever is being studied. It is used in scientific studies to compare with a supposedly active treatment.

Policy Benefits Medical treatments that are covered under a particular health insurance policy.

Positive Thoughts Thoughts that reflect a positive view of reality and help an individual problem solve and cope with difficulties.

Primary Care Doctor A generalist trained in handling a variety of medical problems. A primary care doctor is a family practice doctor or a general internist who rules out serious disease and arrives at a preliminary diagnosis.

Prior Authorization Permission from the health insurance company before receiving treatment. Often required so that the insurance company will pay for treatment.

Prolotherapy Treatment consisting of injections of various chemicals into painful areas.

Pseudarthrosis A condition in which a surgical spine fusion has failed to become solid. *Pseudo* means "false" and *arthro* means "joint."

Psychologically Based Back Pain Pain with no apparent physical reason, requiring mental and/or emotional support to move ahead into progressively more demanding activities.

Psychologist Non-MD professional who helps assess and treat psychosocial needs and behaviors.

Radiculitis Inflammation of a nerve.

Radiculopathy Abnormal functioning of a nerve with nerve pain, with or without neurological deficit.

Radiologist A physician who diagnoses diseases by obtaining and interpreting medical images. Radiologists also treat some diseases by means of radiation or minimally invasive, image-guided surgery.

Referral To send someone to another health care provider, usually a specialist, for more treatment. A doctor's referral is often required by the insurance company.

Referred Pain Pain that is felt in the spine, although the problem itself is not in the spine.

Relaxation Training Tools to induce relaxation in order to decrease stress and muscle tension.

Retrolisthesis A posterior displacement of one vertebra relative to the one below it.

Rolfing A special type of deep muscle massage (see Chapter 3).

Scheuermann's Disease A developmental problem of unknown cause that begins in adolescence and usually has increased kyphosis and pain.

Sciatica Pain in the sciatic nerve. It is most commonly but not always due to disc abnormalities.

Scoliosis A lateral (side-to-side) curvature of the spine with rotation. A normal spine has no scoliosis.

Self-Care What a person does for himself or herself physically and mentally.

Self-Funded Plan A plan in which the employer or group sets aside its own money to pay for health care benefits. States are not allowed to regulate most self-funded plans, thus possibly reducing a person's options for an external review.

Spinal Canal The space inside a vertebra containing the spinal fluid, dural sac, and epidural space (see Chapter 2).

Spinal Stenosis Narrowing of the spinal canal. It is usually associated with compression of the nerves of the cauda equina. There may or may not be neurological deficit.

Spine Neurosurgeon Provides surgical care for disorders of the brain, spinal cord, and nervous system. Tends to perform surgery for tumors of the spinal cord or nerve root, herniated discs, and spinal stenosis (decompression).

Spine Specialist A doctor who may be trained as an orthopedist, neurologist, or physiatrist, the majority of whose patients have back problems.

Spondylolisthesis The slipping forward of one vertebra on another. *Spondy* means "spine" and *olisthesis* means "slipping."

Spondylolysis An area of absent bone in a place where there should be bone. It is most commonly seen in the posterior arch of the fifth lumbar vertebra.

Spondylosis Degenerative changes involving both the discs and facet joints.

SSEP (Somatosensory evoked potential) A test that assesses the speed of electrical conduction along the spinal cord. If the spinal cord is pinched, the electrical signals will travel more slowly than usual. Since the spinal cord ends before the lumbar spine, this test is not used for lumbar spine problems.

Strength Exercises Exercises to build muscle strength and/or mass.

Stress The sum of the biological reactions to any stimulus (the stressor). The stressor is anything physical, mental, emotional, internal, or external that tends to disturb the organism's equilibrium.

Stretching Exercises Exercises that extend a tight or inflexible muscle in order to relax it.

Subluxation Partial dislocation of the vertebrae. This is usually due to major trauma and can be seen on CT or MRI scans.

Summary Plan Description The overview of benefits under a specific health insurance policy.

TENS (Transcutaneous Electrical Nerve Stimulation) The passage of electrical signals through the skin to block the passage of pain signals up to the spinal cord and brain (see Chapter 3).

Therapeutic Exercises Exercises that focus on increasing strength, flexibility, and mobility.

Therapeutic Ultrasoun The use of high-frequency vibrations to effect healing.

Thermotherapy Heat or cold applied locally as a therapeutic agent. Hot packs are used to increase circulation to an area and cold packs are used to diminish pain, especially after exercising.

Torsion Rotation motion of the spine.

Vertebroplasty The technique of placing a large needle into a vertebral body that has a compression fracture. Bone cement or another substance is then injected to stabilize the fracture (see Chapter 4).

Vocational Rehabilitation A service that specializes in helping injured workers return to work. Can help negotiate return to an old job or can help a person learn what jobs are available and the qualifications for those jobs.

Vocational Rehabilitation Specialist Helps with transition back to work or assists in finding a new job that suits physical limitations.

Work Hardening A structured rehabilitation program that uses real or simulated work activities to restore physical and vocational function and is particularly helpful if a person has a physically demanding job or has been out of the workforce for quite some time.

Yoga A series of positioning exercises combined with meditation.

APPENDIX C

References

A Consumer Guide to Handling Disputes with Your Employer or Private Health Plan. Consumers Union, January 2003. www.consumersunion.org/health/hmo-review/.

ACSM's Guidelines for Exercise Testing and Prescription, 6th ed., pp. 171 and 197, Lippincott Williams & Wilkins, Baltimore, 2000.

Agency for Health Care Policy and Research. Choosing a doctor. July 1999.

Ahn N, An H, et al. *Smoking, Smoking Cessation, and Wound Complications After Lumbar Spine Surgery.* Scoliosis Research Society, Seattle, Washington, 2002.

Ahn N, et al. Pain and functional outcomes after IDET: a retrospective review with cost effectiveness. *Spine J* 2003;3:87S.

Albert TJ, Pinto M, Denis F. Management of symptomatic lumbar pseudarthrosis with anteroposterior fusion. A functional and radiographic outcome study. *Spine* 2000;25:123–9; discussion 30.

Alvarez, JA, Hardy, RH. Lumbar spinal stenosis: a common cause of back and leg pain. *American Family Physician* 1998; 57(8):1825–34.

America's obesity crisis. *Time,* pp. 57–113, June 7, 2004.

An H, Jones R, Lynch K. *Prospective Comparison of Autograft Versus Allograft for Spinal Fusion in the Same Patient.* Scoliosis Research Society, Kansas City, 1992.

Assendelft WJ, Koes BW, Knipschild PG, et al. The relationship between methodological quality and conclusions in reviews of spinal manipulation. *JAMA* 1995;274:1942–8.

Assendelft WJ, Morton SC, Yu EI, et al. Spinal manipulative therapy for low back pain. A meta-analysis of effectiveness relative to other therapies. *Ann Intern Med* 2003;138:871–81.

Barrick WT, Schofferman JA, Reynolds JB, et al. Anterior lumbar fusion improves discogenic pain at levels of prior posterolateral fusion. *Spine* 2000; 25:853–7.

Battie MC, Videman T, Gill K, et al. 1991 Volvo Award in clinical sciences. Smoking and lumbar intervertebral disc degeneration: an MRI study of identical twins. *Spine* 1991;16:1015–21.

Battie MC, Videman T, Parent E. Lumbar disc degeneration: epidemiology and genetic influences. *Spine* 2004;29:2679–90.

Bauer HC. Posterior decompression and stabilization for spinal metastases. Analysis of sixty-seven consecutive patients. *J Bone Joint Surg Am* 1997;79: 514–22.

Bello Y, Phillips T. Recent advances in wound healing. *JAMA* 2000; 283(6): 716–8.

Bernstein E, Carey TS, Garrett JM. The use of muscle relaxant medications in acute low back pain. *Spine* 2004;29:1346–51.

Bertagnoli R, Kumar S. Indications for full prosthetic disc arthroplasty: a correlation of clinical outcome against a variety of indications. *Eur Spine J* 2002; 11(suppl 2):S131–6.

Bhatia N, et al. Proximal segment degeneration after posterior lumbosacral fusions (L4-S1 and L5-S1). North American Spine Society, 2002.

Blumenthal SL, Ohnmeiss DD, Guyer RD, et al. Prospective study evaluating total disc replacement: preliminary results. *J Spinal Disord Tech* 2003; 16:450–4.

Boden SD, Davis DO, Dina TS, et al. Abnormal magnetic-resonance scans of the lumbar spine in asymptomatic subjects. A prospective investigation. *J Bone Joint Surg Am* 1990;72:403–8.

Bohlman HH, Zdeblick TA. Anterior excision of herniated thoracic discs. *J Bone Joint Surg Am* 1988;70:1038–47.

Booth KC, Bridwell KH, Eisenberg BA, et al. Minimum 5-year results of degenerative spondylolisthesis treated with decompression and instrumented posterior fusion. *Spine* 1999;24:1721–7.

Boriani S, Biagini R, De Iure F, et al. Primary bone tumors of the spine: a survey of the evaluation and treatment at the Istituto Ortopedico Rizzoli. *Orthopedics* 1995;18:993–1000.

Bradford DS, Schumacher WL, Lonstein JE, et al. Ankylosing spondylitis: experience in surgical management of 21 patients. *Spine* 1987;12:238–43.

Brantigan JW. Pseudarthrosis rate after allograft posterior lumbar interbody fusion with pedicle screw and plate fixation. *Spine* 1994;19:1271–9; discussion 80.

Brantigan JW, Steffee AD, Lewis ML, et al. Lumbar interbody fusion using the Brantigan I/F cage for posterior lumbar interbody fusion and the variable pedicle screw placement system: two-year results from a Food and Drug Administration investigational device exemption clinical trial. *Spine* 2000;25:1437–46.

Bridwell KH, Sedgewick TA, O'Brien MF, et al. The role of fusion and instrumentation in the treatment of degenerative spondylolisthesis with spinal stenosis. *J Spinal Disord* 1993;6:461–72.

Bronfort G, Haas M, Evans RL, Bouter LM. Efficacy of spinal manipulation and mobilization for low back pain and neck pain: a systematic review and best evidence synthesis. *Spine J* 2004;4(3): 335–56.

Brown CW, Orme TJ, Richardson HD. The rate of pseudarthrosis (surgical nonunion) in patients who are smokers and patients who are nonsmokers: a comparison study. *Spine* 1986;11:942–3.

Burkus JK, Lonstein JE, Winter RB, et al. Long-term evaluation of adolescents treated operatively for spondylolisthesis. A comparison of in situ arthrodesis only with in situ arthrodesis and reduction followed by immobilization in a cast. *J Bone Joint Surg Am* 1992;74:693–704.

Burton AK, Clarke RD, McClune TD, et al. The natural history of low back pain in adolescents. *Spine* 1996;21:2323–8.

Buttermann GR, Garvey TA, Hunt AF, et al. Lumbar fusion results related to diagnosis. *Spine* 1998;23:116–27.

Buttermann GR. The effect of spinal steroid injections for degenerative disc disease. *Spine J* 2004;4:495–505.

Button G, Gupta M, et al. Three to six-year follow-up of stand-alone BAK cages implanted by a single surgeon. *Spine J* 2003;3:125S.

Carey TS, Garrett J, Jackman A, et al. The outcomes and costs of care for acute low back pain among patients seen by primary care practitioners, chiropractors, and orthopedic surgeons. The North Carolina Back Pain Project. *N Engl J Med* 1995;333:913–7.

Carey TS, Garrett JM, Jackman A, et al. Recurrence and care seeking after acute back pain: results of a long-term follow-up study. North Carolina Back Pain Project. *Med Care* 1999;37:157–64.

Carr WA, Moe JH, Winter RB, et al. Treatment of idiopathic scoliosis in the Milwaukee brace. *J Bone Joint Surg Am* 1980;62:599–612.

Chappuis J, Corratta C, Orme T. *Simultaneous Circumferential Fusion as an Answer for Multilevel Disease.* North American Spine Society, 1998.

Cherkin DC, Deyo RA, Battie M, et al. A comparison of physical therapy, chiropractic manipulation, and provision of an educational booklet for the treatment of patients with low back pain. *N Engl J Med* 1998;339:1021–9.

Cholewicki J, Alvi K, Silfies SP, et al. Comparison of motion restriction and trunk stiffness provided by three thoracolumbosacral orthoses (TLSOs). *J Spinal Disord Tech* 2003;16:461–8.

Christensen F, Bunger C. Stabilization surgery for chronic low back pain: indications, surgical procedures and outcome. *Scand J Rheumatol* 2004;33:210–7.

Coats TL, Borenstein DG, Nangia NK, et al. Effects of valdecoxib in the treatment of chronic low back pain: results of a randomized, placebo-controlled trial. *Clin Ther* 2004;26:1249–60.

Compliance with physical activity recommendations by walking for exercise— Michigan, 1996 and 1998, Center for Disease Control and Prevention, US Department of Health and Human Services. *Morbidity and Mortality Weekly Report* 2000; 49(25):560–5.

Crandall D, Slaughter D, Hankins PJ, et al. Acute versus chronic vertebral compression fractures treated with kyphoplasty: early results. *Spine J* 2004;4: 418–24.

Crandell, S. Chill out! 23 anti-meltdown tips from the top stress experts. *Prevention* 2005; 57(7):156–67.

Crow NE, Brogdon BG. The normal lumbosacral spine. *Radiology* 1959;72:97.

Currier BL, Eismont FJ, Green BA. Transthoracic disc excision and fusion for herniated thoracic discs. *Spine* 1994;19:323–8.

Danielson BI, Frennered AK, Irstam LK. Radiologic progression of isthmic lumbar spondylolisthesis in young patients. *Spine* 1991;16:422–5.

Davis TT, Delamarter RB, Sra P, et al. The IDET procedure for chronic discogenic low back pain. *Spine* 2004;29:752–6.

Delamarter RB, Fribourg DM, Kanim LE, et al. ProDisc artificial total lumbar disc replacement: introduction and early results from the United States clinical trial. *Spine* 2003;28:S167–75.

Deyo RA, Weinstein JN. Low back pain. *N Engl J Med* 2001;344:363–70.

Diabetes Prevention Program Research Group. The Diabetes Prevention Program (DPP) description of lifestyle intervention. *Diabetes Care* 2002; 25(12): 2165–71.

Dimar JR, 2nd, Campbell M, Glassman SD, et al. Idiopathic juvenile osteoporosis. An unusual cause of back pain in an adolescent. *Am J Orthop* 1995;24: 865–9.

Dreyfuss P, Michaelsen M, Pauza K, et al. The value of medical history and physical examination in diagnosing sacroiliac joint pain. *Spine* 1996;21: 2594–602.

Durr HR, Wegener B, Krodel A, et al. Multiple myeloma: surgery of the spine: retrospective analysis of 27 patients. *Spine* 2002;27:320–4; discussion 5–6.

Early SD, Kay RM, Tolo VT. Childhood diskitis. *J Am Acad Orthop Surg* 2003; 11:413–20.

Edwards CC, Bradford DS. Instrumented reduction of spondylolisthesis. *Spine* 1994;19:1535–7.

Epstein JA, Epstein NE, Marc J, et al. Lumbar intervertebral disk herniation in teenage children: recognition and management of associated anomalies. *Spine* 1984;9:427–32.

Epstein NE. Lumbar synovial cysts: a review of diagnosis, surgical management, and outcome assessment. *J Spinal Disord Tech* 2004;17:321–5.

Errico TJ, Fardon DF, Lowell TD. Open discectomy as treatment for herniated nucleus pulposus of the lumbar spine. *Spine J* 2003;3:45S–9S.

Exercise for patients with coronary heart disease. *American College of Sports Medicine Position Standards,* Medicine & Science in Sports & Exercise, 1994; 26(3):i–v.

Fischgrund JS. The argument for instrumented decompressive posterolateral fusion for patients with degenerative spondylolisthesis and spinal stenosis. *Spine* 2004;29:173–4.

Folman Y, Shabat S, Gepstein R. Relationship between low back pain in postmenopausal women and mineral content of lumbar vertebrae. *Arch Gerontol Geriatr* 2004;39:157–61.

Frazier DD, Campbell DR, Garvey TA, et al. Fungal infections of the spine. Report of eleven patients with long-term follow-up. *J Bone Joint Surg Am* 2001;83-A:560–5.

Freeman BJC, et al. A randomized controlled efficacy study: intradiscal electrothermal therapy (IDET) versus placebo. International Society for Study of the Lumbar Spine (ISSLS). Vancouver, BC, 2003.

Frennered AK, Danielson BI, Nachemson AL. Natural history of symptomatic isthmic low-grade spondylolisthesis in children and adolescents: a seven-year follow-up study. *J Pediatr Orthop* 1991;11:209–13.

Frennered AK, Danielson BI, Nachemson AL, et al. Midterm follow-up of young patients fused in situ for spondylolisthesis. *Spine* 1991;16:409–16.

Fribourg D, Tang C, Sra P, et al. Incidence of subsequent vertebral fracture after kyphoplasty. *Spine* 2004;29:2270–6; discussion 7.

Fritsch EW, Heisel J, Rupp S. The failed back surgery syndrome: reasons, intraoperative findings, and long-term results: a report of 182 operative treatments. *Spine* 1996;21:626–33.

Fritz JM, Delitto A, Welch WC, Erhard RE. Lumbar spinal stenosis: a review of currect concepts in evaluation, management, and outcome measurements. *Arch Phys Med Rehab* 1998: 79:700–8.

Fritzell P, Hagg O, Jonsson D, et al. Cost-effectiveness of lumbar fusion and nonsurgical treatment for chronic low back pain in the Swedish Lumbar Spine Study: a multicenter, randomized, controlled trial from the Swedish Lumbar Spine Study Group. *Spine* 2004;29:421–34; discussion Z3.

Fritzell P, Hagg O, Wessberg P, et al. 2001 Volvo Award Winner in Clinical Studies: lumbar fusion versus nonsurgical treatment for chronic low back pain: a multicenter randomized controlled trial from the Swedish Lumbar Spine Study Group. *Spine* 2001;26:2521–32; discussion 32–4.

Fritzell P, Hagg O, Wessberg P, et al. Chronic low back pain and fusion: a comparison of three surgical techniques: a prospective multicenter randomized study from the Swedish Lumbar Spine Study Group. *Spine* 2002;27: 1131–41.

Frost H, Lamb S. Randomized controlled trial of physiotherapy combined with advice for low back pain. *Brit Med J* 2004;329:708–10.

Gertzbein SD, Hollopeter M, Hall SD. Analysis of circumferential lumbar fusion outcome in the treatment of degenerative disc disease of the lumbar spine. *J Spinal Disord* 1998;11:472–8.

Giles LG, Muller R. Chronic spinal pain: a randomized clinical trial comparing medication, acupuncture, and spinal manipulation. *Spine* 2003;28: 1490–502; discussion 502–3.

Gillet P. The fate of the adjacent motion segments after lumbar fusion. *J Spinal Disord Tech* 2003;16:338–45.

Glassman SD, Anagnost SC, Parker A, et al. The effect of cigarette smoking and smoking cessation on spinal fusion. *Spine* 2000;25:2608–15.

Glassman SD, Minkow RE, Dimar JR, et al. Effect of prior lumbar discectomy on outcome of lumbar fusion: a prospective analysis using the SF-36 measure. *J Spinal Disord* 1998;11:383–8.

Graves N, Krepecho M, Mayo HG. Does yoga speed healing for patients with low back pain? *J Family Practice* 2004;53(8): 661–2.

Grob D, Humke T, Dvorak J. Degenerative lumbar spinal stenosis. Decompression with and without arthrodesis. *J Bone Joint Surg Am* 1995;77:1036–41.

Guide to Health Insurance. America's Health Insurance Plans. 2004. www.ahip.org/content/default.aspx?bc=41;vb329;vb351.

Guyer RD, Ohnmeiss DD. Lumbar discography. *Spine J* 2003;3:11S–27S.

Hambly MF, Wiltse LL, Raghavan N, et al. The transition zone above a lumbosacral fusion. *Spine* 1998;23:1785–92.

Hanley EN, Jr., David SM. Lumbar arthrodesis for the treatment of back pain. *J Bone Joint Surg Am* 1999;81:716–30.

Hansen F, Biering-Sorensen F, Schroll M. MMPI profiles in persons with or without low back pain: a 20-year follow-up study. *Spine* 1995;20:2716–20.

Harrington KD. Metastatic disease of the spine. *J Bone Joint Surg Am* 1986;68: 1110–5.

Harris GR, Susman JL. Managing musculoskeletal complaints with rehabilitation therapy: summary of the Philadelphia Panel evidence-based clinical practice guidelines on musculoskeletal rehabilitation interventions. *J Family Practice* 2002; 51(12):1042–7.

Haughton V. Medical imaging of intervertebral disc degeneration: current status of imaging. *Spine* 2004;29:2751–6.

Hee HT, Castro FP, Jr., Majd ME, et al. Anterior/posterior lumbar fusion versus transforaminal lumbar interbody fusion: analysis of complications and predictive factors. *J Spinal Disord* 2001;14:533–40.

Hefti F, Seelig W, Morscher E. Repair of lumbar spondylolysis with a hook-screw. *Int Orthop* 1992;16:81–5.

Heithoff KB, Gundry CR, Burton CV, et al. Juvenile discogenic disease. *Spine* 1994;19:335–40.

Herkowitz HN. Spine update. Degenerative lumbar spondylolisthesis. *Spine* 1995; 20:1084–90.

Herkowitz HN, Kurz LT. Degenerative lumbar spondylolisthesis with spinal stenosis. A prospective study comparing decompression with decompression and intertransverse process arthrodesis. *J Bone Joint Surg Am* 1991;73:802–8.

Herron LD, Mangelsdorf C. Lumbar spinal stenosis: results of surgical treatment. *J Spinal Disord* 1991;4:26–33.

Herzog RJ, Ghanayem AJ, Guyer RD, et al. Magnetic resonance imaging: use in patients with low back pain or radicular pain. *Spine J* 2003;3:6S–10S.

Hilibrand AS, Rand N. Degenerative lumbar stenosis: diagnosis and management. *J Am Acad Orthop Surg* 1999;7:239–49.

Hinkley BS, Jaremko ME. Effects of 360-degree lumbar fusion in a workers' compensation population. *Spine* 1997;22:312–22; discussion 23.

How to be a smart patient, *U.S. News & World Report,* pp. 47–63, November 8, 2004.

Hsieh CY, Adams AH, Tobis J, et al. Effectiveness of four conservative treatments for subacute low back pain: a randomized clinical trial. *Spine* 2002; 27:1142–8.

Hurley DA, McDonough SM, Dempster M, et al. A randomized clinical trial of manipulative therapy and interferential therapy for acute low back pain. *Spine* 2004;29:2207–16.

Iwane M, et al. Walking 10,000 steps/day or more reduces blood pressure and sympathetic nerve activity in mild essential hypertension, *Hypertension Res* 2000;23(6):573–80.

Jensen MC, Brant-Zawadzki MN, Obuchowski N, et al. Magnetic resonance imaging of the lumbar spine in people without back pain. *N Engl J Med* 1994;331:69–73.

Johnsson KE, Uden A, Rosen I. The effect of decompression on the natural course of spinal stenosis. A comparison of surgically treated and untreated patients. *Spine* 1991;16:615–9.

Johnsson KE, Willner S, Johnsson K. Postoperative instability after decompression for lumbar spinal stenosis. *Spine* 1986;11:107–10.

Jorgenson SS, Lowe TG, France J, et al. A prospective analysis of autograft versus allograft in posterolateral lumbar fusion in the same patient. A minimum of 1-year follow-up in 144 patients. *Spine* 1994;19:2048–53.

Just say om, *Time,* pp. 48–56, August 4, 2003.

Kaila-Kangas L, Leino-Arjas P, Riihimaki H, et al. Smoking and overweight as predictors of hospitalization for back disorders. *Spine* 2003;28:1860–8.

Kambin P. Arthroscopic microdiscectomy. *Spine J* 2003;3:60S–4S.

Katz JN, Lipson SJ, Chang LC, et al. Seven- to 10-year outcome of decompressive surgery for degenerative lumbar spinal stenosis. *Spine* 1996;21:92–8.

Katz N, Ju WD, Krupa DA, et al. Efficacy and safety of rofecoxib in patients with chronic low back pain: results from two 4-week, randomized, placebo-controlled, parallel-group, double-blind trials. *Spine* 2003;28:851–8; discussion 9.

Kemmler W, Lauber D, Weineck J, et al. Benefits of 2 years of intense exercise on bone density, physical fitness, and blood lipids in early postmenopausal osteopenic women: results of the Erlangen Fitness Osteoporosis Prevention Study (EFOPS). *Arch Intern Med* 2004;164:1084–91.

Kimura I, Shingu H, Murata M, et al. Lumbar posterolateral fusion alone or with transpedicular instrumentation in L4–L5 degenerative spondylolisthesis. *J Spinal Disord* 2001;14:301–10.

King HA. Evaluating the child with back pain. *Pediatr Clin North Am* 1986;33: 1489–93.

Koes BW, Assendelft WJ, van der Heijden GJ, et al. Spinal manipulation for low back pain. An updated systematic review of randomized clinical trials. *Spine* 1996;21:2860–71; discussion 72–3.

Koes BW, Bouter LM, van Mameren H, et al. A randomized clinical trial of manual therapy and physiotherapy for persistent back and neck complaints:

subgroup analysis and relationship between outcome measures. *J Manip Physiol Ther* 1993;16:211–9.

Koes BW, van Tulder MW, Ostelo R, et al. Clinical guidelines for the management of low back pain in primary care: an international comparison. *Spine* 2001;26:2504–13; discussion 13–4.

Kornblum MB, Fischgrund JS, Herkowitz HN, et al. Degenerative lumbar spondylolisthesis with spinal stenosis: a prospective long-term study comparing fusion and pseudarthrosis. Spine 2004;29:726–33; discussion 33–4.

Kwon BK, Berta S, Daffner SD, et al. Radiographic analysis of transforaminal lumbar interbody fusion for the treatment of adult isthmic spondylolisthesis. J Spinal Disord Tech 2003;16:469–76.

Lagrone MO, Bradford DS, Moe JH, et al. Treatment of symptomatic flatback after spinal fusion. *J Bone Joint Surg Am* 1988;70:569–80.

Lauerman WC, Bradford DS, Ogilvie JW, et al. Results of lumbar pseudarthrosis repair. *J Spinal Disord* 1992;5:149–57.

Laurent LE, Einola S. Spondylolisthesis in children and adolescents. *Acta Orthop Scand* 1961;31:45–64.

Lehmer SM, Steffee AD, Gaines RW, Jr. Treatment of L5-S1 spondyloptosis by staged L5 resection with reduction and fusion of L4 onto S1 (Gaines procedure). *Spine* 1994;19:1916–25.

Le Masurier G, Sidman C, Corbin C. Accumulating 10,000 steps: does this meet current physical activity guidelines? *Res Q Exercise Sport* 2003;74(4): 389–94.

Letts M, Haasbeek J. Hematocolpos as a cause of back pain in premenarchal adolescents. *J Pediatr Orthop* 1990;10:731–2.

L'Heureux EA, Jr., Perra JH, Pinto MR, et al. Functional outcome analysis including preoperative and postoperative SF-36 for surgically treated adult isthmic spondylolisthesis. *Spine* 2003;28:1269–74.

Licciardone JC, Stoll ST, Fulda KG, et al. Osteopathic manipulative treatment for chronic low back pain: a randomized controlled trial. *Spine* 2003;28: 1355–62.

Liddle SD, Baxter GD, Gracey JH. Exercise and chronic low back pain: what works? *Pain* 2004; 107(1–2): 176–90.

Lifeso RM, Weaver P, Harder EH. Tuberculous spondylitis in adults. *J Bone Joint Surg Am* 1985;67:1405–13.

Long A, Donelson R, Fung T. Does it matter which exercise? A randomized control trial of exercise for low back pain. *Spine* 2004;29:2593–602.

Lonstein JE, Winter RB. The Milwaukee brace for the treatment of adolescent idiopathic scoliosis. A review of one thousand and twenty patients. *J Bone Joint Surg Am* 1994;76:1207–21.

Louisia S, Anract P, Babinet A, et al. Long-term disability assessment after surgical treatment of low grade spondylolisthesis. *J Spinal Disord* 2001;14: 411–6.

Lowe TG. Scheuermann disease. *J Bone Joint Surg Am* 1990;72:940–5.

Lowe TG, Tahernia AD, O'Brien MF, et al. Unilateral transforaminal posterior lumbar interbody fusion (TLIF): indications, technique, and 2-year results. *J Spinal Disord Tech* 2002;15:31–8.

MacDonald PB, Black GB, MacKenzie R. Orthopedic manifestations of blastomycosis. *J Bone Joint Surg Am* 1990;72:860–4.

MacDougall JB, Perra JH, Pinto MR. Incidence of adjacent segment degeneration at 10 years after lumbar spine fusion. North American Spine Society, 2003.

Malcolm BW, Bradford DS, Winter RB, et al. Post-traumatic kyphosis. A review of forty-eight surgically treated patients. *J Bone Joint Surg Am* 1981;63: 891–9.

Mardjetko SM, Connolly PJ, Shott S. Degenerative lumbar spondylolisthesis. A meta-analysis of literature 1970–1993. *Spine* 1994;19:2256S–65S.

Maruta T, Colligan R, Malinchoc M, Offord K. Optimists vs. pessimists: survival rate among medical patients over a 30-year period. *Mayo Clin Proc* 2000;75:140–3.

Mathews JA, Mills SB, Jenkins VM, et al. Back pain and sciatica: controlled trials of manipulation, traction, sclerosant and epidural injections. *Br J Rheumatol* 1987;26:416–23.

Matsunaga S, Sakou T, Morizono Y, Masuda A, Demirtas AM. Natural history of degenerative spondylolisthesis—pathogenesis and natural history of slippage. *Spine* 1990; 15(11): 1204–10.

Mayer T, McMahon MJ, Gatchel RJ, et al. Socioeconomic outcomes of combined spine surgery and functional restoration in workers' compensation spinal disorders with matched controls. *Spine* 1998;23:598–605; discussion 6.

Mayer T, Polatin P, Smith B, et al. Spine rehabilitation: secondary and tertiary nonoperative care. *Spine J* 2003;3:28S–36S.

Mazzotta MY. Nutrition and wound healing. *J Am Podiatr Med Assoc* 1994; 84(9): 456–62.

McKenzie RA. *The Lumbar Spine. Mechanical Diagnosis and Therapy.* Spinal Publications Limited, Waikanae, New Zealand, 1981.

Meditation: tuning the mind to help heal the body. *Mayo Clin Health Lett* 2005;23(3):4–5.

Moller H, Hedlund R. Surgery versus conservative management in adult isthmic spondylolisthesis—a prospective randomized study: part 1. *Spine* 2000;25: 1711–5.

Moore KR, Pinto MR, Butler LM. Degenerative disc disease treated with combined anterior and posterior arthrodesis and posterior instrumentation. *Spine* 2002;27:1680–6.

Mulkana SS, Hailey BJ.N. The role of optimism in health-enhancing behavior. *Am J Health Behav* 2001;25(4): 388–95.

Mullin BB, Rea GL, Irsik R, et al. The effect of postlaminectomy spinal instability on the outcome of lumbar spinal stenosis patients. *J Spinal Disord* 1996;9:107–16.

Murray PM, Weinstein SL, Spratt KF. The natural history and long-term follow-up of Scheuermann kyphosis. *J Bone Joint Surg Am* 1993;75:236–48.

Nachemson A. Recent advances in the treatment of low back pain. *Int Orthop* 1985;9:1–10.

Nachemson AL. Proceedings: treatment of low back pain: a critical look at current methods. *J Bone Joint Surg Br* 1975;57:262.

Nachemson AL, Peterson LE. Effectiveness of treatment with a brace in girls who have adolescent idiopathic scoliosis. A prospective, controlled study based on data from the Brace Study of the Scoliosis Research Society. *J Bone Joint Surg Am* 1995;77:815–22.

National Institutes of Health. Clinical guidelines on the identification, evaluation, and treatment of overweight and obesity in adults—the evidence report. *NIH Pub. No. 98-4083.* National Heart, Lung and Blood Institute, Bethesda, MD, 1998; 228 pages. See also *Obes Res* 1998;6(suppl 2):51S–209S.

Nelson ME, Fiatorone MA, Morganti CM et al. Effects of high-intensity strength training on multiple risk factors for osteoporotic fracture. *JAMA* 1994; 272:1909–14.

Nibu K, Panjabi MM, Oxland T, et al. Multidirectional stabilizing potential of BAK interbody spinal fusion system for anterior surgery. *J Spinal Disord* 1997;10:357–62.

Nicol RO, Scott JH. Lytic spondylolysis. Repair by wiring. *Spine* 1986;11: 1027–30.

Niemeyer T, Bovingloh AS, Halm H, et al. Results after anterior-posterior lumbar spinal fusion: 2–5 years follow-up. *Int Orthop* 2004;28:298–302.

Niemisto L, Lahtinen-Suopanki T, Rissanen P, et al. A randomized trial of combined manipulation, stabilizing exercises, and physician consultation compared to physician consultation alone for chronic low back pain. *Spine* 2003;28:2185–91.

Nork SE, Hu SS, Workman KL, et al. Patient outcomes after decompression and instrumented posterior spinal fusion for degenerative spondylolisthesis. *Spine* 1999;24:561–9.

Nyiendo J, Haas M, Goldberg B, et al. Pain, disability, and satisfaction outcomes and predictors of outcomes: a practice-based study of chronic low back pain patients attending primary care and chiropractic physicians. *J Manip Physiol Ther* 2001;24:433–9.

O'Beirne J, O'Neill D, Gallagher J, et al. Spinal fusion for back pain: a clinical and radiological review. *J Spinal Disord* 1992;5:32–8.

O'Brien JP, Dawson MH, Heard CW, et al. Simultaneous combined anterior and posterior fusion. A surgical solution for failed spinal surgery with a brief review of the first 150 patients. *Clin Orthop* 1986:191–5.

O'Dowd J, Lam K, Mulholland R, et al. *The Bagby and Kuslich Cage: The Nottingham Results of a Prospective, Non-Randomized Study.* North American Spine Society, 1998.

O'Sullivan PB, Twomey LT, Allison GT. Evaluation of specific stabilizing exercises in the treatment of chronic low back pain with radiologic diagnosis of spondylolysis or spondylolisthesis. *Spine* 1997;22(24): 2959–67.

Ottenbacher K, DiFabio RP. Efficacy of spinal manipulation/mobilization therapy. A meta-analysis. *Spine* 1985;10:833–7.

Ozerdemoglu RA, Denis F, Transfeldt EE. Scoliosis associated with syringomyelia: clinical and radiologic correlation. *Spine* 2003;28:1410–7.

Patwardhan A, et al. Relaxation response of lumbar segments undergoing disc-space distraction: implications to the stability of stand-alone anterior lumbar interbody implants. Scoliosis Research Society. Buenos Aires, Argentina, 2004.

Pauza KJ, Howell S, Dreyfuss P, et al. A randomized, placebo-controlled trial of intradiscal electrothermal therapy for the treatment of discogenic low back pain. *Spine J* 2004;4:27–35.

Pedometers. *Consumer Reports,* pp. 30–31, October 2004.

Pellise F, Puig O, Rivas A, et al. Low fusion rate after L5-S1 laparoscopic anterior lumbar interbody fusion using twin stand-alone carbon fiber cages. Spine 2002;27:1665–9.

Pettine KA, Klassen RA. Osteoid-osteoma and osteoblastoma of the spine. *J Bone Joint Surg Am* 1986;68:354–61.

Phillips FM, Ho E, Campbell-Hupp M, et al. Early radiographic and clinical results of balloon kyphoplasty for the treatment of osteoporotic vertebral compression fractures. *Spine* 2003;28:2260–5; discussion 5–7.

Picavet HS, Schuit AJ. Physical inactivity: a risk factor for low back pain in the general population? *J Epidemiol Community Health* 2003;57:517–8.

Pilowsky I. Low back pain and illness behavior (inappropriate, maladaptive, or abnormal). *Spine* 1995;20:1522–4.

Pinto J, Whitecloud T, et al. Transforaminal lumbar interbody fusion for the treatment of degenerative conditions of the lumbar spine. *Spine J* 2003;3: 1085–95.

Pizzutillo PD, Hummer CD, 3rd. Nonoperative treatment for painful adolescent spondylolysis or spondylolisthesis. *J Pediatr Orthop* 1989;9:538–40.

Pollock et al. Effects of frequency and duration of training on attrition and incidence of injury. *Med Sci Sports Exercise* 1977;9:31–6.

Pope MH, Phillips RB, Haugh LD, et al. A prospective randomized three-week trial of spinal manipulation, transcutaneous muscle stimulation, massage and corset in the treatment of subacute low back pain. *Spine* 1994;19:2571–7.

Postacchini F. Surgical management of lumbar spinal stenosis. *Spine* 1999;24: 1043–7.

Pradham B, Delamarter R, Dawson E, et al. Can rh BMP-2 (InFuse) enhance fusion rates in anterior lumbar interbody fusion using stand-alone femoral ring allografts? Scoliosis Research Society. Buenos Aires, Argentina, 2004.

Preparing for Surgery, Johns Hopkins Family Health Book, Klag MJ, ed., pp. 1427–46, HarperCollins, New York, 1999.

Pre-surgery and post-surgery instructions, Online/University of Pittsburgh Medical Center Website, http://patienteducation.upmc.com/S.htm#Surgery.

Rafferty AP, et al. Physical activity patterns among walkers and compliance with public health recommendations. *Med Sci Sports Exercise* 2002;34(8): 1255–61.

Rahm MD, Hall BB. Adjacent-segment degeneration after lumbar fusion with instrumentation: a retrospective study. *J Spinal Disord* 1996;9:392–400.

Ramirez N, Johnston CE, Browne RH. The prevalence of back pain in children who have idiopathic scoliosis. *J Bone Joint Surg Am* 1997;79:364–8.

Rating the diets from Atkins to Zone, *Consumer Reports,* pp. 18–22, June 2005.

Robertson PA, Jackson SA. Prospective assessment of outcomes improvement following fusion for low back pain. *J Spinal Disord Tech* 2004;17:183–8.

Rowe DE, Bernstein SM, Riddick MF, et al. A meta-analysis of the efficacy of non-operative treatments for idiopathic scoliosis. *J Bone Joint Surg Am* 1997;79:664–74.

Sachs B, Bradford D, Winter R, et al. Scheuermann kyphosis. Follow-up of Milwaukee-brace treatment. *J Bone Joint Surg Am* 1987;69:50–7.

Saifuddin A, White J, Sherazi Z, et al. Osteoid osteoma and osteoblastoma of the spine. Factors associated with the presence of scoliosis. *Spine* 1998;23: 47–53.

Salminen JJ, Erkintalo M, Laine M, et al. Low back pain in the young. A prospective three-year follow-up study of subjects with and without low back pain. *Spine* 1995;20:2101–7; discussion 8.

Salminen JJ, Erkintalo MO, Pentti J, et al. Recurrent low back pain and early disc degeneration in the young. *Spine* 1999;24:1316–21.

Sanderson PL, Wood PL. Surgery for lumbar spinal stenosis in old people. *J Bone Joint Surg Br* 1993;75:393–7.

Saraste H. Long-term clinical and radiological follow-up of spondylolysis and spondylolisthesis. *J Pediatr Orthop* 1987;7:631–8.

Sasso RC, Kitchel SH, Dawson EG. A prospective, randomized controlled clinical trial of anterior lumbar interbody fusion using a titanium cylindrical threaded fusion device. *Spine* 2004;29:113–22; discussion 21–2.

Schlenzka D, Poussa M, Seitsalo S, et al. Intervertebral disc changes in adolescents with isthmic spondylolisthesis. *J Spinal Disord* 1991;4:344–52.

Schnitzer TJ, Ferraro A, Hunsche E, et al. A comprehensive review of clinical trials on the efficacy and safety of drugs for the treatment of low back pain. *J Pain Symptom Manage* 2004;28:72–95.

Schwender JD, Denis F, Garvey TA, et al. Revision lumbar arthrodesis for the treatment of cylindrical cage pseudoarthrosis: perioperative complications and pitfalls. North American Spine Society, Seattle, 2001.

Schwender J, Ogilvie J. Prospective study of the cantilever TLIF: radiographic and patient outcomes with minimum two-year follow-up. *Spine J* 2003;3: 1095.

Seitsalo S, Osterman K, Hyvarinen H, et al. Progression of spondylolisthesis in children and adolescents. A long-term follow-up of 272 patients. *Spine* 1991;16:417–21.

Shaw M, Birch N. Facet joint cysts causing cauda equina compression. *J Spinal Disord Tech* 2004;17:442–5.

Shaw JM, Witzke KA. Exercise for skeletal health and osteoporosis prevention. *ACSM's Resource Manual for Guidelines for Exercise Testing and Prescription,* 3rd ed., pp. 288–93, Lippincott Williams and Wilkings, Baltimore, 1998.

Shekelle PG, Adams AH, Chassin MR, et al. Spinal manipulation for low-back pain. *Ann Intern Med* 1992;117:590–8.

Seigel RD, Urdang MH, Johnson DR. *Back Sense*, pp. 149–150, Broadway Books, New York, 2001.

Silcox DH, 3rd, Daftari T, Boden SD, et al. The effect of nicotine on spinal fusion. *Spine* 1995;20:1549–53.

Simmons ED, Guyer RD, Graham-Smith A, et al. Radiograph assessment for patients with low back pain. *Spine J* 2003;3:3S–5S.

Sinaki M, Wollan PC, Scott RW, Gelcer RK. Can strong back extensors prevent vertebral fractures in women with osteoporosis? *Mayo Clin Proc* 1997; 71(10):951–6.

Sinel MS, Deardorff WW. *Back Pain Remedies for Dummies*, pp. 243–54, IDG Books Worldwide, Inc., Foster City, CA, 1999.

Skargren EI, Carlsson PG, Oberg BE. One-year follow-up comparison of the cost and effectiveness of chiropractic and physiotherapy as primary management for back pain. Subgroup analysis, recurrence, and additional health care utilization. *Spine* 1998;23:1875–83; discussion 84.

Slosar PJ, Reynolds JB, Schofferman J, et al. Combined anterior and posterolateral lumbar fusions: primary and revision procedures. North American Spine Society, 1994.

Slosar PJ, Reynolds JB, Schofferman J, et al. Patient satisfaction after circumferential lumbar fusion. *Spine* 2000;25:722–6.

Smith BW, Zautra AJ. The role of purpose in life in recovery from knee surgery. *Int J Behav Med* 2004;11(4):197–202.

Smith EL, Gilligan C, Kwiatkowski BS. Osteoporosis: background and management, Lewis CB, Knortz KA, eds. *Orthopedic Assessment and Treatment of the Geriatric Patient*, pp. 395–410, Mosby-Year Book, Inc., St. Louis, MO, 1993.

Smith-Petersen MN, Larson CB, Aufranc OE. Osteotomy of the spine for correction of flexion deformity in rheumatoid arthritis. *Clin Orthop* 1969;66:6–9.

Snider RK, Krumwiede NK, Snider LJ, et al. Factors affecting lumbar spinal fusion. *J Spinal Disord* 1999;12:107–14.

Sobel, DS, Mind matters, money matters: the cost effectiveness of mind/body medicine. *JAMA* 2000;284(13):1705.

Spivak JM. Current concepts review of degenerative lumbar spinal stenosis. *J Bone Joint Surg* 1998:80(7):1053–66.

Stokes IA, Iatridis JC. Mechanical conditions that accelerate intervertebral disc degeneration: overload versus immobilization. *Spine* 2004;29:2724–32.

Swenson R, Haldeman S. Spinal manipulative therapy for low back pain. *J Am Acad Orthop Surg* 2003;11:228–37.

Tachdjian MO, Matson DD. Orthopedic aspects of intraspinal tumors in infants and children. *J Bone Joint Surg Am* 1965;47:223–48.

Taimela S, Kujala UM, Salminen JJ, et al. The prevalence of low back pain among children and adolescents. A nationwide, cohort-based questionnaire survey in Finland. *Spine* 1997;22:1132–6.

Taking Charge of Your Health Care, Johns Hopkins Family Health Book, Klag MJ, ed., pp. 1383–426, HarperCollins, New York, 1999.

Tamaya-Orozco J, Arzac-Palumbo P, Peon-Vidales H, Mota-Bolfeta R, Fuente F. Vertebral fractures associated with osteoporosis: patient management. *Am J Med* 1997;103(2A):44–50.

Tay BK, Deckey J, Hu SS. Spinal infections. *J Am Acad Orthop Surg* 2002;10: 188–97.

Taylor ME. Return to work following back surgery: a review. *Am J Ind Med* 1989;16(1):79–88.

Taylor RS, Van Buyten JP, Buchser E. Spinal cord stimulation for chronic back and leg pain and failed back surgery syndrome: a systematic review and analysis of prognostic factors. *Spine* 2005;30:152–60.

Thomasen E. Vertebral osteotomy for correction of kyphosis in ankylosing spondylitis. *Clin Orthop* 1985:142–52.

Tribus CB. Scheuermann's kyphosis in adolescents and adults: diagnosis and management. *J Am Acad Orthop Surg* 1998;6:36–43.

Tribus CB. Degenerative lumbar scoliosis: evaluation and management. *J Am Acad Orthop Surg* 2003;11:174–83.

Trowbridge CA, Draper DO, Feland JB, et al. Paraspinal musculature and skin temperature changes: comparing the Thermacare HeatWrap, the Johnson & Johnson Back Plaster, and the ABC Warme-Pflaster. *J Orthop Sports Phys Ther* 2004;34:549–58.

Tsou PM, Yeung C, Yeung AT. Posterolateral transforaminal selective endo-scopic discectomy and thermal annuloplasty for chronic lumbar discogenic pain: a minimal access visualized intradiscal surgical procedure. *Spine J* 2004;4:564–73.

Tudor-Locke C, Bassett DR. How many steps/day are enough? Preliminary pe-dometer indices for public health. *Sports Med* 2004;34(1):1–8.

Tudor-Locke C, et al. Descriptive epidemiology of pedometer determined phys-ical activity. *Med Sci Sports Exercise* 2004;36(9):1567–73.

Udermann BE, Spratt KF, Donelson RG, et al. Can a patient educational book change behavior and reduce pain in chronic low back pain patients? *Spine J* 2004;4:425–35.

Understanding Your Spine Surgery, 2nd ed., Allina Hospitals and Clinics, Al-lina Health System Press, 2002.

Vanichkachorn JS, Vaccaro AR. Thoracic disk disease: diagnosis and treatment. *J Am Acad Orthop Surg* 2000;8:159–69.

van Tulder MW, Koes BW, Bouter LM. Conservative treatment of acute and chronic nonspecific low back pain. A systematic review of randomized controlled trials of the most common interventions. *Spine* 1997;22:2128–56.

Verbeek J, Sengers MJ, Riemens L, et al. Patient expectations of treatment for back pain: a systematic review of qualitative and quantitative studies. *Spine* 2004;29:2309–18.

Waddell G. 1987 Volvo Award in clinical sciences. A new clinical model for the treatment of low-back pain. *Spine* 1987;12:632–44.

Wand BM, Bird C, McAuley JH, et al. Early intervention for the management of acute low back pain: a single-blind randomized controlled trial of biopsychosocial education, manual therapy, and exercise. *Spine* 2004;29:2350–6.

Wang JM, Kim DJ, Yun YH. Posterior pedicular screw instrumentation and anterior interbody fusion in adult lumbar spondylolysis or grade I spondylolisthesis with segmental instability. *J Spinal Disord* 1996;9:83–8.

Wang SM, Dezinno P, Maranets I, et al. Low back pain during pregnancy: prevalence, risk factors, and outcomes. *Obstet Gynecol* 2004;104:65–70.

Weber H. Spine update: the natural history of disc herniation and the influence of intervention. *Spine* 1994;19(19):2234–8.

Weiner BK, Fraser RD. Spine update lumbar interbody cages. *Spine* 1998;23:634–40.

Weiner DK, Ernst E. Complementary and alternative approaches to the treatment of persistent musculoskeletal pain. *Clin J Pain* 2004;20:244–55.

Weinstein JN, McLain RF. Primary tumors of the spine. *Spine* 1987;12:843–51.

Weinstein SM, Herring SA. Lumbar epidural steroid injections. *Spine J* 2003;3:37S–44S.

Wenger DR, Frick SL. Scheuermann kyphosis. *Spine* 1999;24:2630–9.

Wilson E, Payton O, Donegan-Shoaf L, Dec K. Muscle energy technique in patients with acute low back pain: a pilot clinical trial. *J Orthop Sports Phys Ther* 2003;33(9):502–12.

Wiltse LL, Radecki SE, Biel HM, et al. Comparative study of the incidence and severity of degenerative change in the transition zones after instrumented versus noninstrumented fusions of the lumbar spine. *J Spinal Disord* 1999;12:27–33.

Wiltse LL, Widell EH, Jr., Jackson DW. Fatigue fracture: the basic lesion is isthmic spondylolisthesis. *J Bone Joint Surg Am* 1975;57:17–22.

Wiltse LL, Winter RB. Terminology and measurement of spondylolisthesis. *J Bone Joint Surg Am* 1983;65:768–72.

Winter R. Congenital scoliosis: approach and treatment. *Semin Spine Surg* 1997;9:80–96.

Winter RB. Congenital spine deformity: What's the latest and what's the best? *Spine* 1989;14:1406–9.

Winter RB, Schellhas KP. Painful adult thoracic Scheuermann's disease. Diagnosis by discography and treatment by combined arthrodesis. *Am J Orthop* 1996;25:783–6.

Yelland MJ, Del Mar C, Pirozzo S, et al. Prolotherapy injections for chronic low back pain: a systematic review. *Spine* 2004;29:2126–33.

Yelland MJ, Glasziou PP, Bogduk N, et al. Prolotherapy injections, saline injections, and exercises for chronic low-back pain: a randomized trial. *Spine* 2004;29:9–16; discussion.

Your Guide to Choosing Quality Health Care. September 2002. Agency for Health Care Policy and Research. www.ahrq.gov/consumer/qntascii/qntcover.htm.

Zdeblick TA. A prospective, randomized study of lumbar fusion. Preliminary results. *Spine* 1993;18:983–91.

Zigler JE. Clinical results with ProDisc: European experience and U.S. investigation device exemption study. *Spine* 2003;28:S163–6.

Index

Page numbers in *italics* refer to illustrations.

abdominal curls, 244, *244*
  on an exercise ball, 255, *255*
  with weights, 249, *249*
abdominal muscles, 12
abdominal sets, 201, *201*
abdominal wall, *14*
acetaminophen (Tylenol), 8, 40, 41
active extension exercise, 45
active flexion exercise, 45
active lateral bending, 45
active torsion (oblique
  strengthening), 45
acupuncture, 51, *55*
acute back pain, 18, 100–101, 136,
  137, 188
addiction, narcotic, 40, 42, 43, 75,
  131
adolescents, *See* children.
Advil (ibuprofen), 8, 40, 41, 44
aerobic exercise, 260–66
  See also walking
aging, 22, 24
Aleve (naproxen sodium), 8, 41, 44,
  93
ALIF, *See* anterior lumbar
  interbody fusion.
alkaline phosphatase, 89
allergic reactions, 40, 54
all four arm and leg lift, 248, *248*

allograft, 60–61
alternative treatments, insurance
  coverage of, 147
American Academy of Family
  Practice, 106
American Academy of Orthopedic
  Surgeons, 106
American Association of
  Neurological Surgeons, 107
American Board of Medical
  Specialties, 128
American Board of Orthopedic
  Surgery, 93
American College of Surgeons,
  134
American Medical Massage
  Association, 48–49
Americans with Disabilities Act,
  160
ankle pumps, 200, *200*, 211
ankylosing spondylitis, 33, 65,
  139–40
annular tear, *19*
annulus fibrosis, 11–12, *13*, 17, *19*,
  20, 60, 63
anterior discectomy, 58–60
anterior interbody fusion and
  posterolateral fusion with
  instrumentation, 64, 278

anterior lumbar fusion:
    with cylindrical cage, 62, 278–79
    with strut graft, 62
anterior lumbar interbody fusion
        (ALIF):
    with bone graft, 60–61, *61*, 279
    with stand-alone cage, 61
anterior thoracic fusion:
    with cylindrical cage, 62
    with strut grafts, 62
antibiotics, 34, 140
antiinflammatory medications, 8,
        41–42, 44, 70
arm lift on an exercise ball, 253, *253*
arthritis, 24, 42
artificial disc replacement, 66–67,
        67
artificial discs, 23, 67
artificial ligaments, 68
aspirin, 8, 40, 41
autografts, 60, 68
automatic thinking, 213–16
    benefits of, 214–15
    changing negative to positive in,
        215–16

Bach, Marilyn L., 86–98
back:
    developing a healthy, 237–75
    strengthening of, 4, 242–60
    uniqueness of individual, 2
    See also spine
back brace, 23, 26, 50–51, 55, 209
    for children, 284
    for recreational sports, 266, 267
    types of, 51
Back Care Pyramid, 98–99, 100,
        125–35, 196

acute back pain level of, 137
based on evidence-based
        medicine, 125
chronic back pain level of, 138
family doctor as second step on,
        127–28, 132
physicians on, 127–32
self-care as first step on, 126
specialists as third step on,
        128–30
spine specialists as fourth step on,
        129–30
spine surgeons as fifth step on,
        130–31
subacute pain level of, 137
back education:
    as part of physical therapy,
        170–71, 173–74
    See also posture and position
back pain:
    advice from others about, 82
    best websites on, 106–8
    causes of, 3, 15–35, 100–101
    as common ailment, 1, 7
    diagnosis of, *see* diagnosis
    healing tools for, 3
    less common causes of, 33–35
    most common questions about,
        70–76
    nonspine causes of, 35
    as primarily benign, 9
    psychological causes of, 34, 287
    as symptom vs. diagnosis, 136
    treatments for, *see* treatments
    when to seek medical help for, 9
    as workplace injury, 153
bedside manner, 135
bending, *see* lifting and bending

Benson, Herbert, 220
Bextra, 44
biking, stationary biking, 265–66
biofeedback training, 220
biopsy, 34
bladder, 35, 71
block tests, 120, 124
blood clotting, 41
blood transfusion, 204–5
body mass index (BMI), 271–72
body mechanics, 45, 233–34
body's natural healing, 38, 42
bone density, 27, 28
bone grafts, 60–61, 68
bone metabolism, 50
bone scan, 34, 122, 286
Botox, 74
bowels, 35, 71
bowling, 268
brace, *see* back brace
breast reduction surgery, 16
breathing exercises, 203, 211, 217,
    218
bulging disc, *19*
buttock squeeze, 201, *201*

calcium, 50, 73
calories, 273–74
cancer, back pain due to, 34,
    285–86
capsular ligaments, *13*
carbamazepine (Tegretol), 44
cardiovascular fitness, *see* aerobic
    exercise
carisoprodol (Soma), 42
cars, getting in and out of, 230
cartilage, 42
catheter, 211

CAT (computerized axial
    tomography) scan, 89, 122
cauda equina syndrome, 17
Celebrex, 44, *95*
central stenosis, 23, 25
cervical vertebrae, 10, *11*
chair position, 235
chair push-ups, 201, *201*
Charite, 66
chemonucleolysis, 54, *55*
chemotherapy, 33, 34, 286
chest, 12
    See also thoracic spine
children:
    back pain in, 3, 282–87
    gynecological source of back pain
        in, 287
    premature disc degeneration in,
        284–85
    psychological vs. physical causes
        of back pain in, 282, 287
    Scheuermann's disease in,
        283–84
    scoliosis in, 32, 51, 285
    spinal bone tumors in, 286
    spinal cord tumors in, 285–86
    spinal infections in, 287
    spondylolysis and
        spondylolisthesis in, 282–83
chiropractics, 7, 45–46, 139
    as controversial, 45
    effectiveness of, 46, 101
    evidence in support of, 46
    insurance coverage of, 46, 147
    subluxation manipulation as basis
        of, 45–46
    training in, 45
chondroitin sulfate, 42

chronic back pain, 103, 136
    choosing treatment for, 138–40
    depression due to, 52, 115
    as non-diagnosis, 113
    surgical treatments for, 69
chronic pain clinics, 280
circulatory system, 109
codeine, 18, 43
    Tylenol with, 43, 95
commercial websites, 107–8
computed tomography (CT) scan,
        16, 27, 122, 283
computerized axial tomography
        (CAT) scan, 89, 122
computer position, 235
congenital scoliosis, 31
contour position, 8, 8, 18
copay, 148
copper bracelets, 53, 55
cortisone, 33, 95
coughing:
    as breathing exercise, 203, 211
    fragility fractures caused by, 27
Cox-2 inhibitors, 44
C-reactive protein, 120
cryotherapy, 74
CT myelogram, 27, 123, 279
CT (computed tomography) scans,
        16, 27, 122, 283
cyclobenzaprine (Flexeril), 42

Darvocet, 95
Darvon (propoxyphene), 43
Darvon Compound, 43
decompression operations, 56–60,
        59, 96–97, 131, 191, 277, 278
deep breathing exercises, 199, 203,
        211, 217, 218

degenerative scoliosis, 31, 31, 51
degenerative spondylolisthesis,
        25–27, 94, 122
    accompanied by spinal stenosis,
        27
    treatment for, 26–27
Demerol (meperidine), 18, 43
depression, 18, 52, 115, 206
desk position, 235
diagnosis:
    challenging of, 89, 115
    ensuring accuracy of, 115–16
    by family doctor, 109, 110–11,
        127, 137
    missed or delayed, 114, 276–77
    understanding of, 3, 89
diagonal abdominal curl, 245, 245
    on an exercise ball, 256, 256
    with weights, 250, 250
dietitians, 209
Dilaudid (hydromorphone), 44
disability, going on, 232
disc degeneration, 21–23, 21, 24,
        94, 115
    causes of, 22, 72, 73–74
    degenerative scoliosis due to,
        30–31, 31
    degenerative spondylolisthesis
        caused by, 26
    familial tendency to, 72
    fusion operation as cause of,
        73–74
    physical therapy for, 177, 189
    premature, in children, 284–85
    progression of, 73
    symptoms of, 22
    treatments for, 22–23, 139, 177,
        189

discectomy, 58–60, 72, 277
discogram, 123
discs, 11–12, *13*
    artificial, 23, 66–67, *67*
    degeneration of, *see* disc
        degeneration
    herniation of, *see* herniated discs
    lumbar spine, *19*
    torn, 72
double knee to chest stretch, 240,
    240
dressing after surgery, 206, 227–28,
    227, 228
Drug Enforcement Administration
    (DEA), 43
dura, 69
Duragesic (fentanyl patch), 44

education:
    about back, 170–71, 173–74
    and making informed decisions,
        83–84
    and self-care, 92
    about specialties, 133–34
    about treatments, 92–93, 115
EKG (electrocardiogram), 88
elective treatments, insurance
    coverage of, 147
electrocardiogram (EKG), 88
electrodiagnostic tests, 123–24
electromyogram, electromyography
    (EMG), 123, 185
empowerment, 79, 198–99
endoscopic decompression, 60
enteric coated aspirin, 41
epidural abscess, 34
epidural steroid injections, 25, 26,
    47, 54, 73, 75, 189

ergonomics, 170–71
evidence-based medicine, 36–39
    Back Care Pyramid based on, 125
    physical therapy, 173–74
exercise:
    disciplined approach to, 173
    learning about, 171, 173
    as part of self-care, 102
    as physical therapy tool, 45,
        92–93, 164, 171–72
    presurgical, 199–203
    soreness from, 179
    for spine stabilization, 22, 23, 45
    as treatment for disc
        degeneration, 22
    in treatment of spondylolysis and
        spondylolisthesis, 26, 30
    see also strengthening program;
        stretching program; *specific*
        exercises
exercise ball, 45, 94
    abdominal curls on, 255, *255,*
        256, 256
    arm lift on, 253, *253*
    leg extension on, 248, *248*
    leg lifts, 258, *258*
    one leg squat with, 259, *259*
    two leg squat with, 254, *254*
experimental treatments, insurance
    coverage of, 147
Explanation of Medicare Benefits
    form, 151
extensor muscles, 12, *14*
external review organizations,
    (EROs), 159–60

facet block tests, 124
facet joints, 12, *13,* 24, 26, 29, 62

facet rhizotomy, 54, 55
falling, 16, 100
family doctor, 7, 109–18
  diagnosis made by, 109, 110–11,
    127, 137
  duration of treatment by, 128, 138
  failure to heed patient by, 114
  follow-ups with, 89
  as initial medical contact, 87–88,
    92, 98, 109
  openness with, 110
  referrals from, 88, 93, 109, 112,
    127, 128, 138
  as second step on Back Care
    Pyramid, 127–28, 132
  selection of, 112–13, 147–48
  tests ordered by, 111
  what to expect from examination
    by, 110–12
fentanyl patch (Duragesic), 44
First Report of Injury form, 153
Flexeril (cyclobenzaprine), 42
flexor muscles, in contour
  position, 8
Food and Drug Administration
  (FDA), 23, 44, 66, 147
foramen, 23, 57, 59
foraminae, 15, 24
foraminal decompression, 58
foraminal stenosis, 23, 25, 59
fortitude, 80, 81
fragility fractures, 27
fusion operations, 23, 57, 60–66,
  61, 63, 115, 191, 283
  for degenerative spondylolisthesis,
    26–27
  disc degeneration caused by, 73–74
  motion abilities after, 73–74

osteoporosis and recovery from,
    74–75
  recovery from, 73, 74–75, 277,
    278; see also surgical
    treatments, recovery from
  removal of instrumentation after,
    75
  smoking as hindrance to healing
    after, 72, 278
  see also specific operations
fusion with bone morphogenetic
  protein (BMP), 66

gabapentin (Neurontin), 44
Gary, 114
general rehabilitation physicians, see
  physiatrists
Gloria, 114–15
glucosamine, 42
golf, 267–68
golfer's lift, 228, 228
guided imagery, 221
gynecological problems, back pain
  due to, 35, 112, 287

half-kneel lift, 229, 234, 299
hamstring stretch, 239, 239
Hatha yoga, 50
health care directive, 204
health care team:
  hospital affiliations of, 134, 164,
    188
  right mindset for meeting with,
    78, 80–81, 169, 209
  for surgical treatments, 208–9
  trust and working with, 83
health insurance provider, 1, 3,
    141–62

appeals process of, 157–60
contact before treatment with,
   152–54, 204
independent rating agencies for,
   144
keeping record of contact with,
   154–55
key principles of, 142–43
legal action against, 160
ombudsperson at, 117
and payment of duplicate
   benefits, 149–50
profit motives of, 142
referral services from, 182
resolving conflicts with, 155–60
through work, 144
see also insurance policy
health maintenance organizations
   (HMOs), 146
healthy eating, 203–4, 223, 237,
   268–75
heat or hot packs, 172
application of, 8, 45, 70, 223
herniated discs treated with, 18,
   101
herniated discs, 122
causes of, 17, 19, 20
in children, 287
physical therapy for, 176–77
progression of, 74
self-care for, 18
symptoms of, 17
treatment of, 17–18, 47, 72, 101,
   131, 176–77, 279
hip flexor stretch, 241, 241
hips, 8, 12, 14
HIV, 33
hospital referral service, 182

hospital stay, 207–12
health care team during, 208–9
ins and outs of, 210–12
pain management during,
   209–10, 211
visitors during, 206
house, preparations for post-op
   return to, 205–6
hydrocodone (Vicodin), 43
hydromorphone (Dilaudid), 44
hypnosis, 220–21

ibuprofen (Advil; Motrin), 8, 40,
   41, 44, 93, 94
ice or cold packs, 172, 223
application of, 8, 18, 45, 70,
   101
IDET (intradiscal
   electrothermography), 54, 55
idiopathic scoliosis, 30–31
braces in treatment of, 51
in children, 285
imaging tests, 120–23
immune system, spinal infections
   and, 33
indemnity insurance policy, 145–46,
   147
insurance policy:
chiropractics covered by, 46, 147
exclusions in coverage from,
   146–47
home health care covered by, 91
indemnity vs. managed care,
   145–46
massage covered by, 49, 147
patient costs under, 149
physical therapy covered by, 45,
   147, 165–66

insurance policy: (*continued*)
  physicians covered by, 91, 134,
    147–48
  post-op costs and, 207
  questions about coverage by,
    143–52
  referrals covered by, 148
  second opinions covered by,
    117–18, 145
  selection of doctor and, 113,
    147–48
  specialists covered by, 91, 144,
    184
  surgical procedures not covered
    by, 66
  understanding of, 142–52
  who to ask about, 152
intercostal muscles, 15
internal disc derangement, *19*
internal review, at health insurance
    provider, 157–59
Internet, 104–8
interspinous spacers, 68
intradiscal electrothermography
    (IDET), 54, *55*
intramuscular injections, 210
intrathecal medications, 210
intravenous medications, 210
Iowa, University of, 107
isometrics, 45
isthmic spondylolisthesis, 29–30,
    29, 139
isthmic spondylolysis, 29–30, *29*,
    68

job, *see* work
joint degeneration, medications for,
    42

joint mobilizations, 172
*Journal of the American Academy
    of Orthopedic Surgery,* 46

kidneys, kidney stones, 35, 109, 112
knees, in contour position, *8*
knee to chest stretch, 240, *240*
kyphoplasty, 28, 67
kyphosis, *11*, 32, 279, 283

laboratory tests, 119–20
Labor Department, U.S., 160
laminae, *24, 29, 58, 62, 68*
laminectomy, 25, 63, 69, 72, 278,
    280
  with foraminotomy, 25
  and spinal canal decompression,
    58, 59
laminotomy, 72
laparoscopic surgery, 88
Learned Optimism (Seligman), 80
legal action, against insurance
    providers, 160
leg extension on an exercise ball,
    248, *248*
leg lifts on an exercise ball, 258,
    258
legs, back pain as origin of problem
    with, 71, 92, 277
level one appeal (desk review), 158
level two appeal, 159
lifting and bending, 92
  avoidance of, 39–40, 70, 100,
    101
  correct way of, 170
  herniated discs caused by, 17, 18
  muscle strain or ligament sprain
    from, 16

spinal fractures and, 27
after surgery, 224, 228–29, 233–34
ligaments, 12, *13*
enlargement of, 24
sprains and, 16, 287
ligamentum flavum, *13, 58*
liver damage, 41, 89–92
log rolls, 201
lordosis, *11, 13*
lower back, *see* lumbar spine
lumbar disc herniation, 58, 60
lumbar hemilaminotomy and disc fragment removal, 58
lumbar lordosis, 65
lumbar posterolateral fusion, 62, *62*
with instrumentation, 62–63, *63*
lumbar roll, 93
lumbar spine, 12, *13, 14, 29*
discs in, *19*
nerves in, *15*
vertebrae in, 11, *11, 24, 63*

McKenzie, Robin, 93
McKenzie school of exercises, 171
magnetic resonance imaging (MRI), 16, 17, 27, 34, 96, 121–22, 139, 279, 283, 285, 286, 287
magnets, 53, *55*
managed care insurance policy, 145–46, 147–48
see also insurance policy
manual techniques, 45
massage, 45, 48–49, 55, 172
as complementary treatment, 48, 147
training in, 48–49
massage recliner chairs, 53, 55

Mayo Clinic, 91, 107
Healthy Weight Pyramid from, 268–70, *269*
Mayo Clinic: Healthy Weight for Every Body, 270
Medicaid, 150–51, 152
medical decisions:
comfort level with, 196–97
education and, 83–84
taking charge of, 90, 91, 92–98
Medicare, 150–51, 152
Medicare Advantage program, 150
Medicare Secondary Payer (MSP), 150
Medicare Summary Notice, 151
medications, 40–44
allergy role in selection of, 40
best, for back pain, 70
effectiveness of, 54, 139
for herniated discs, 18
for osteoporosis prevention, 28
side effects of, 40
before surgery, 197–98
testing of, 40
see also over-the-counter medications; pain medications; *specific medications*
meditation, 217, 220
mental and emotional health:
physical connection to, 213–21
for return to work, 233
self-care and, 40, 101, 225
See also psychotherapy
mental imagery, 217, 218–19, 223, 233
meperidine (Demerol), 18, 43
metastatic cancer, back pain due to, 34

methocarbamol (Robaxin), 42
microdiscectomy, 58
Mind-Body Connection, The
    (Sarno), 51
mini-squats, 201
mobility exercises, 173
morphine, 18, 44
morphine pump, 69, 280, 281
motor nerves, 15
Motrin (ibuprofen), 40, 41
MRI, *See* magnetic resonance
    imaging.
multifidi, 12
muscle energy techniques (METs),
    172
muscle relaxants, 42
muscles, *14*
    pilates and, 49
    spine movement controlled by, 12
    strengthening exercises for, 171,
        242–60
    tightening of, 82–83, 199
    weakness in, 15
muscle spasms, 42
muscle strain, 16
    causes of, 16
    physical therapy for, 175–76
    symptoms of, 16
    treatment of, 16
myelogram, 122
myofascial release, 48

Naprosyn (naproxen), 41, 44
naproxen sodium (Aleve), 8, 41, 44,
    93
Narco, 43
narcotics, 280
    for herniated discs, 18

    risk of addiction to, 40, 42, 43,
        75, 131
National Committee For Quality
    Assurance, (NCQA), 144
National Institutes of Health (NIH),
    108
neck, vertebrae in, *See* cervical
    vertebrae.
nerve conduction tests, 124, 185
nerve root blocks, 47, 55, 124
nerve root decompression, 25, 131,
    277, 278
nerves, pinched, 71
neurologists, 129–30, 132
Neurontin (gabapentin), 44
neurosurgeons, 7, 131, 132, 187,
    190, 191, 286
nonsteroidal antiinflammatory
    drugs (NSAIDs), 41, 44, 70
nonsurgical treatments, 36–55, 139
    for degenerated discs, 22–23
    effectiveness of, 1, 7, 54–55
    for herniated discs, 18
    surgical treatments avoided or
        delayed by, 47
    See also specific treatments
North American Spine Society,
    106–7
NSAIDs, *See* nonsteroidal
    antiinflammatory drugs.
nucleus pulposis, *19, 20*
nurse, nurse practitioner (NP),
    127–28, 208

obliques, external and internal, 12,
    14
occupational therapists, 209
one-leg bridging, 251, *251*

one-leg bridging with ankle
weights, 256, *256*
one leg squat with an exercise ball,
259, *259*
optimism, 79–80, 81, 223
orthopedic surgeons or specialists, 7,
93–98, 128–29, 130, 132, 187
questions for, 93–94
referrals from, 129
scope of practice of, 128–29
training of, 128
orthotist, 209
osteoarthritis, 94
osteoid osteoma, 286
osteoporosis, 27
aggravated by smoking, 28, 71
physical therapy for, 177
prevention of, 28, 50, 73
recovery from fusion operation
with, 74–75
spine fractures and, 27–28, 67
osteotomy, 65–66
over-the-counter (OTC) medications,
8, 22, 40–42, 101
oxycodone (Oxycontin; Percodan),
18, 44, 95

pacing, 233, 235
pain medications:
effectiveness of, 111
during hospital stay, 209–10
OTC, 41
prescription, 42–44
for Scheuermann's Disease, 32
See also narcotics
Pandiscio, Cate, 97
paralysis, from thoracic disc
herniation, 17

pars interarticularis repair, 68
patient-controlled analgesia (PCA)
pump, 210
patient passivity, 87–92
patient's rights, 198–99
pedicles, 24, *63*, 65
pedicle screws, 68
pedicle subtraction osteotomy and
refusion, 65–66
pedometer walking program,
261–64
pelvis, 11, *11*, *14*, 67
Percocet, 43
Percodan (oxycodone), 43
peritoneum, 89, 90
Perra, Joseph, 93–94, 95, 96–97
physiatrists, 129, 132, 183–87
checking out, 184
first visit to, 184–85
referrals from, 129, 186
selecting of, 187
with spinal speciality, 130,
132
treatments used by, 186
physical medicine and rehabilitation
(PM&R), 129, 183, 185–86,
187
physical therapists, 7, 22, 92, 93,
164, 209, 211
defined, 163–64
duration and frequency of visits
to, 165
examination and evaluation by,
168–69
first visit to, 168–69
hands-on techniques of, 172
interpersonal skills of, 167
patient evaluation by, 164

physical therapists (*continued*)
  program designed by, 164, 173
  referrals to, 92, 165–66
  selecting of, 166–68
  with spinal specialty, 116, 166, 167
  training and background of, 163, 167
  traits of a good, 167–68
physical therapy, 94, 139, 170–79
  back education and, 170–71
  continuity of care as key in, 167
  diagnosis-specific, 175–78
  effectiveness of, 45, 54, 174
  evidence-based, 173–74
  exercise as tool of, 164, 171–72
  home program for, 173
  modalities of, 45, 164, 172–73
  pain during, 178–79
  pilates and, 49, 92, 93
  postoperative, 91, 97, 178
  presurgical, 96, 178
  for Scheuermann's disease, 32, 44–45
physicians:
  on Back Care Pyramid, 127–32
  bedside manner of, 135
  checking credentials of, 133–34
  degrees held by, 133
  experience of, 134–35
  health insurance coverage of, 134
  questions for, 83, 88, 90, 96, 111, 134–35
  referrals from and for, 88, 92, 93, 95, 109, 112, 113
  selecting of, 2, 3, 84, 88, 92
  specialties of, 133–34
physician's assistant (PA), 127, 128

pilates, 49, 55, 92, 93
Pinto, Manuel, 76
piriformis stretch, 242, *242*
placebo effect, 37
PLIF (posterior lumbar interbody fusion), 63
PM&R, *See* physical medicine and rehabilitation.
point-of-service (POS) plans, 146
posterior fusion mass osteotomy and refusion, 65
posterior instrumentation and fusion for spinal deformity, 64, 67, 279
posterior lumbar interbody fusion (PLIF), 63
posture and position, 45, 71, 75, 165, 211, 223–24, 233–36
  muscle strain due to, 16
  in sitting or standing, 102, 234, 235–36
  in sleeping, 93, 230
  training for, 45, 170, 234–35
preferred provider organizations (PPOs), 146
premiums, insurance, 143
prescription drug benefits (Part D of Medicare), 150
prescription medications, 42–44
press-up, 241, *241*
primary-care doctor, *See* family doctor.
prolotherapy, 54, 55
propoxyphene (Darvon), 43
pseudarthrosis, 278, 279
psoas, 12
psychotherapy, 51–52, 55, 280, 281, 286

PubMed (National Institutes of Health website), 108

quadratus lumborum, 12

racquet sports, 266
radiation, 34, 121, 286
radiculopathy, 94
radiofrequency, 74
radiologists, 25
recreational sports, participating safely in, 266–68
rectus abdominus, 12
referred pain, 112
rehabilitation centers, after surgery, 207
rehabilitation physicians, *See* physiatrists.
relaxation exercises and techniques, 199, 210, 217–21, 223
Relaxation Response, The (Benson), 220
rheumatoid arthritis, 33
rhizotomy, 74
ribs, 67–68
right mindset, 77–85
  about advice from others, 82
  in dealing with insurance provider, 156
  defined, 77–79
  for meeting with health care team, 78, 80–81, 169, 209
  in self-care, 40, 101, 225
  and surgery, 196–97, 198–99, 223, 225, 280
  tips for, 83–85
Robaxin (methocarbamol), 42
rolfing, 48

running, 265
ruptured discs, *see* herniated discs
Russell, Eve, 92, 93, 95, 96

sacrum, 11, *11, 13, 29*
Sarno, John, 34, 51–52
Scheuermann's disease, 32, 72, 115
  causes of, 32
  in children, 283–84
  symptoms of, 32
  treatment of, 32, 51, 178
  See also kyphosis
scoliosis, 30–32, *30, 31*
  causes of, 30–31, 287
  in children, 32, 51, 285
  symptoms of, 31
  treatment of adults with, 31, 51, 67–68, 178
Scoliosis Association, Inc., 107
Scoliosis Research Society, 107
second opinions, 94
  after failed surgery, 280
  insurance coverage of, 117–18, 145
  before surgical treatments, 193–94, 197
sedimentation rate, 120
self-care, 3, 7–8, 9, 39–40, 100–103, 287
  emotional health in, 40, 101, 225
  as first step on Back Care Pyramid, 126
  in listening to body, 84
  OTC medications and, 40
Seligman, Martin, 80
sensory nerves, 15
sequestered disc, *20*
serum protein analysis, 120

sexual activity, post-op, 225
showering and bathing, after
    surgery, 205, 228
side-lying leg lift, 247, *247*
side-lying leg lift with an exercise
    band, 257, *257*
side-lying leg lift with rotation, 252,
    252
sitting posture, 223, 234, 235–36
sleep, posture and position during,
    93, 223, 230
Smith-Petersen osteotomy, 65
smoking, 237
    healing hampered by, 39, 71,
        102, 224
    osteoporosis linked to, 28, 72
    pre-surgical restrictions on, 198
Social Security Act, 150
social workers, 209
soft tissue mobilization, 172
Soma (carisoprodol), 42
somatosensory evoked potential
    (SSEP), 185
spasms, from herniated discs, 18
special beds, 52, *55*
specialists:
    on Back Pain Pyramid, 98–99
    examination by, 138–39
    getting appointment with, 182–83
    meeting and working with, 180–92
    in physical therapy, 97
    referrals to, 109, 112, 127, 128,
        138, 181–82
    surgeons referred from, 95
    surgical treatments by, 90–91
    as third step on Back Care
        Pyramid, 128–30
    types of, 128–30

See also spine specialists; spine
    surgeons
spinal bone tumors, and back pain
    in children, 286
spinal canal, *20*, 23, *24*, 58, 122
spinal cord, 15, 17, 23, 57, 131
spinal cord stimulation, 69, 280
spinal cord tumors, 285–86
spinal infections, 33–34, 140, 287
spinal nerves, *13*, 15, 17, *20*, 23, 57
spinal stenosis, 23–25, 71, 122, 277
    accompanied by degenerative
        spondylolisthesis, 27
    causes of, 24
    physical therapy for, 175
    recurrence of, 279
    symptoms of, 25
    treatment of, 25, 47, 58, *59*, 72,
        75, 131
spine:
    in contour position, *8*
    structure and function of, 10–15,
        11
    See also back; lumbar spine;
        thoracic spine
spine fractures:
    braces in treatment of, 50
    osteoporosis-related, 27–28
spine specialists, 187–90
    checking out, 188
    first visit to, 188–89
    as fourth step on Back Care
        Pyramid, 129–30
    selecting of, 190
    treatments used by, 90–91, 189
    types of, 129–30
spine stabilization exercises, 22, 23,
    45

spine surgeons, 139, 190–94, 208
  in consultation after failed
    surgery, 280
  as fifth step on Back Care
    Pyramid, 130–31
  first visit to, 192–93
  need for surgery determined by,
    192
  orthopedic vs. neurological, 190,
    191
  recommendation for surgery
    from, 193–94
  referrals from family doctor to,
    88, 93
  referrals from specialists to, 95
  selecting of, 192
  types of, 130–31
spondylolisthesis
  in children, 282–83
  degenerative, 25–27, 94, 122,
    176
  isthmic, 29–30, 29, 139
spondylolysis:
  in children, 282–83
  isthmic, 29–30, 29, 68
spurs, 21, 24, 24, 25
standing posture, 234–35
stomach ulcers, 41
strengthening program, 171, 173,
    242–60, 260
  level one, 243–48
  level two, 249–54
  level three, 255–60
stress, 216–21
  lowering of, 217–18
  negative thoughts and, 214
  relaxation exercises for, 199,
    210, 217–21

tightened muscles due to, 82–83,
    199
stretching program, 45, 171, 173,
    238–42
subacute back pain, 100–102, 136,
    188
  choosing the right treatment for,
    137–38
  with herniated disc, 18
  self-care of, 102
surgical treatments, 56–69
  avoiding aspirin before, 41
  blood transfusion for, 204–5
  for central stenosis, 25
  comfort level and, 196–97
  for degenerated discs, 23
  for disc herniation, 17, 18
  failure of, 276–81
  follow-up meeting before, 84, 88,
    139–40
  for foraminal stenosis, 25
  getting second opinions before,
    193–94, 197
  hospital stay for, 207–12
  of isthmic spondylolysis and
    spondylolisthesis, 30, 68
  and lower back pain, 76
  mental preparation for, 198–99
  night and morning before, 207–8
  for osteoporosis-related spine
    fractures, 28
  physical examination before,
    197–98
  physical preparation for,
    199–204
  physical therapy and, 91, 96, 97,
    178
  preparing for successful, 195–212

surgical treatments (*continued*)
  put off by nonsurgical treatments,
    47, 94
  questions to ask about, 88, 90,
    96, 192–93, 196–97
  for Scheuermann's Disease, 32
  secondary problems caused by,
    279
  setting date for, 197
  time off work required for, 197
  *See also specific types of surgical
    treatments*
surgical treatments, recovery from:
  at-home support, 206–7, 223, 224
  expectations about, 222–30
  follow-ups, 89
  gradual increase in activities in,
    211, 225
  pain management and, 211,
    223–24
  resumption of daily activities in,
    227–30
  return home in, 205–6
  return to work in, 231–36
  self-care in, 224–25
  transitional care unit, 207
  walking, *see* walking program,
    post-op
Swedish massage, 48
swimming, 264
synovial facet joint cyst, 33
syringomyelia, 287

Tegretol (carbamazepine), 44
TENS (transcutaneous electrical nerve
    stimulation) units, 53, 55, 74
tests, 111, 119–24
  See also specific tests

thigh squeeze, 200, *200*
thoracic disc herniation, 17, 58–60
thoracic spine:
  nerves in, 15
  vertebrae of, 11, *11*
thoracoplasty, 67–68
TLIF (transforaminal lumbar
    interbody fusion), 63
touch therapy, 48
traction, 53, 55, 173
tramadol (Ultram), 43
transcutaneous electrical nerve
    stimulation (TENS) units, 53,
    55, 74
transforaminal lumbar interbody
    fusion (TLIF), 63
transitional care unit, after surgery,
    207
transversalis muscles, 12, *14*
trauma:
  from falls, 16, 100
  muscle strain or ligament sprain
    from, 16
  spinal fractures caused by, 27
treatments:
  effectiveness of, 1, 7, 111
  evidence-based medicine and,
    36–39
  most common questions about,
    70–76
  patient as active partner in, 83
  payers for, 152–53
  selecting of, 1–2, 136–40
  self-administered, *see* self-care
  See also nonsurgical treatments;
    surgical treatments
Treat Your Own Back (McKenzie),
    93

tuberculosis, 287
two-leg bridging, 246, *246*
two-leg lift, 229, *229*, 234
two-leg squat with an exercise ball, 254, *254*
Tylenol (acetaminophen), 8, 40, 41
    #3 and # 4 (with codeine), 43, *95*
Tylot, 43

Ultram (tramadol), 43
ultrasound, 45
university medical centers, as information sources, 107

vertebrae, 10–11, *13, 62*
    cervical, 10, *11*
    lumbar, 11, *11, 24, 63*
    slippage of, 25–26
    thoracic spine, 11, *11*
vertebroplasty, 28, 67
Vicodin (hydrocodone), 43
Vicodin ES, 43
Vicoprophen, 43
Vioxx, 44
Vitamin D, 50
vitamins, 50, *55*
vocational training, 232

walking, 22, *95*
    counting steps and, 262
    gait examination and, 11
    as ideal aerobic exercise, 261–64
    increasing step count for, 263

and pain prevention, 39
    setting goals for, 262–63
    spinal stenosis aggravated by, 25
    as treatment for disc degeneration, 22, 94
walking program, post-op, 97, 211, 226–27
Washington, University of, 107
water exercise, 22, 102
Web MD Health Site, 107
weight:
    determining healthy, 271–72
    healing hindered by excess, 39, 102, 271
weight lifting, 266–67
weight loss, 272–75
Williams school of exercises, 171
work, injury from, 153
work, returning to:
    good body mechanics in, 233–34
    office set up for, 235–36
    posture and position in, 234–36
    preparing for, 233
    restrictions on, 231
    after surgery, 231–36
worker's compensation, 153
work hardening, 232

X-rays, 16, 34, 120–23, 139, 283, 286

yoga, 49–50, *55*

WANT TO LIVE WELL?

LIVING WELL WITH MIGRAINE DISEASE AND HEADACHES
What Your Doctor Doesn't Tell You . . . That You Need to Know
by Teri Robert, Ph.D.
0-06-076685-9 (trade paperback)
A holistic, patient-centered guide to the diagnosis, side effects and treatments for headaches and Migraine disease.

LIVING WELL WITH MENOPAUSE
What Your Doctor Doesn't Tell You . . . That You Need To Know
by Carolyn Chambers Clark, ARNP, Ed.D.
0-06-075812-0 (trade paperback)
A complete holistic guide and self-care manual to menopause.

LIVING WELL WITH HYPOTHYROIDISM
What Your Doctor Doesn't Tell You . . . That You Need to Know
by Mary J. Shomon
0-06-074095-7 (trade paperback)
An expanded and updated edition of the hugely successful *Living Well with Hypothyroidism*.

LIVING WELL WITH GRAVES' DISEASE AND HYPERTHYROIDISM
What Your Doctor Doesn't Tell You . . . That You Need to Know
by Mary J. Shomon
0-06-073019-6 (trade paperback)
Here is a holistic road map for diagnosis, treatment, and recovery from Graves' disease and hyperthyroidism.

LIVING WELL WITH EPILEPSY AND OTHER SEIZURE DISORDERS
An Expert Explains What You Really Need to Know
by Carl W. Bazil. M.D., Ph.D
0-06-053848-1 (trade paperback)
A much-needed book of information, support, and lifestyle strategies for this surprisingly common problem.

LIVING WELL WITH ENDOMETRIOSIS
What Your Doctor Doesn't Tell You . . . That You Need to Know
by Kerry-Ann Morris
0-06-084426-4 (trade paperback)
A complete guide to the side effects and treatments—both conventional and alternative—for endometriosis.

LIVING WELL WITH CHRONIC FATIGUE SYNDROME AND FIBROMYALGIA
What Your Doctor Doesn't Tell You . . . That You Need to Know
by Mary J. Shomon
0-06-052125-2 (trade paperback)
A comprehensive guide to the diagnosis and treatment of chronic fatigue syndrome and fibromyalgia.

LIVING WELL WITH AUTOIMMUNE DISEASE
What Your Doctor Doesn't Tell You . . . That You Need to Know
by Mary J. Shomon
0-06-093819-6 (trade paperback)
A complete guide to understanding the mysterious disorders of the immune system.

LIVING WELL WITH ANXIETY
What Your Doctor Doesn't Tell You . . . That You Need to Know
by Carolyn Chambers Clark, ARNP, Ed.D.
0-06-082377-1 (trade paperback)
A complete guide to the side effects and treatments for anxiety disorders.

Visit www.AuthorTracker.com
for exclusive information on your favorite HarperCollins authors.

Available wherever books are sold, or call 1-800-331-3761 to order.